Clinicians' Guide

Clinicians' Guide to Angina

Edited by

Michael J. Walsh MD FRCPI FRCP FESC FACC
Consultant Cardiologist, St James's Hospital,
Dublin, Ireland, and Associate Professor,
Cardiology, Trinity College, Dublin, Ireland

Emer Shelley MD MSc FRCPI FFPHM FFPHMI
National Heart Health Advisor,
Department of Health and Children, Dublin, Ireland,
and Lecturer in Epidemiology, Royal College of Surgeons in
Ireland, Dublin, Ireland

and

Ross T. Murphy MD MRCPI
Specialist Registrar in Cardiology, St George's Hospital
Medical School, London, UK

ARNOLD

A member of the Hodder Headline Group
LONDON

First published in Great Britain in 2003 by
Arnold, a member of the Hodder Headline Group,
338 Euston Road, London NW1 3BH

http://www.arnoldpublishers.com

Distributed in the USA by
Oxford University Press Inc.,
198 Madison Avenue, New York, NY10016
Oxford is a registered trademark of Oxford University Press

Whilst the advice and information in this book are believed to be true and accurate at the date of going to press, neither the author[s] nor the publisher can accept any legal responsibility or liability for any errors or omissions that may be made. In particular (but without limiting the generality of the preceding disclaimer) every effort has been made to check drug dosages; however, it is still possible that errors have been missed. Furthermore, dosage schedules are constantly being revised and new side-effects recognized. For these reasons the reader is strongly urged to consult the drug companies' printed instructions before administering any of the drugs recommended in this book.

British Library Cataloguing in Publication Data
A catalogue record for this book is available from the British Library

Library of Congress Cataloging-in-Publication Data
A catalog record for this book is available from the Library of Congress

ISBN 0 340 80671 0

1 2 3 4 5 6 7 8 9 10

Commissioning Editor: Joanna Koster
Production Editor: Wendy Rooke
Production Controller: Bryan Eccleshall
Cover Designer: Terry Griffiths

Typeset in 11/13pt Adobe Garamond by Charon Tec Pvt. Ltd, Chennai, India
Printed and bound in Malta by Gutenberg Press Ltd

What do you think about this book? Or any other Arnold title?
Please send your comments to feedback.arnold@hodder.co.uk

Contents

List of contributors

Dr Michael Barry
National Centre for
Pharmacoeconomics
St James's Hospital
Dublin, Ireland

Dr Peter Crean
Consultant Cardiologist
CResT Directorate
St James's Hospital
Dublin, Ireland

Professor John Feely
Department of Pharmacology and
Therapeutics
Trinity College
Dublin, Ireland

Dr J. Brendan Foley
Consultant Cardiologist
CResT Directorate
St James's Hospital
Dublin, Ireland

Dr Gerard Gearty
Consultant Cardiologist
CResT Directorate
St James's Hospital
Dublin, Ireland

Dr Robert Kelly
Specialist Registrar in Cardiology
CResT Directorate
St James's Hospital
Dublin, Ireland

Dr Eilis McGovern
Consultant Cardiothoracic Surgeon
CResT Directorate
St James's Hospital
Dublin, Ireland

Dr Geraldine McMahon
Consultant in Emergency Medicine
St James's Hospital
Dublin, Ireland

Professor Andrew W. Murphy
Department of General Practice
National University of Ireland
Galway, Ireland

Dr Ross T. Murphy
Department of Cardiological
Sciences
St George's Hospital Medical
School
London, UK

Dr Emer Shelley
National Heart Health Advisor
Department of Health and Children
Dublin, Ireland, and
Lecturer in Epidemiology
Royal College of Surgeons in Ireland
Dublin, Ireland

Professor Michael J. Walsh
Consultant Cardiologist
CResT Directorate
St James's Hospital
Dublin, Ireland, and
Associate Professor, Cardiology
Trinity College
Dublin, Ireland

Foreword

Angina pectoris is the mode of presentation of half of all patients with ischaemic heart disease. Contrary to popular belief, myocardial infarction accounts for only about one-sixth of patients presenting for the first time, sudden death a quarter and the remainder have unstable angina. Ischaemic heart disease is, of course, the most important cause of death in the Western world. Governments have now begun to understand the importance of this condition and are pouring enormous resources into its management. However, the management of angina, unlike almost any other condition, differs dramatically from country to country, depending principally on resources but also on the enthusiasm of cardiologists and the availability of invasive facilities. Sometimes this enthusiasm may ignore current available evidence and thus it is important for those training in cardiology to have available a sensible, straightforward approach to this condition. Every doctor in the world practising medicine will see patients with angina on a daily basis and, indeed, it will be for many the bread and butter of their clinical practice. Michael Walsh, Emer Shelley and Ross Murphy have, together with their colleagues in Dublin, prepared a text in straightforward and simple style. The text is comprehensive, covering as it does the epidemiology, pathophysiology, clinical diagnosis and investigation as well as medical, interventional and surgical treatment. It concludes with the enormous health economic aspects of this condition. Boxes are used to highlight salient features, and figures and tables liberally supplement the text. Finally, in a field as rapidly advancing as coronary disease, this book keeps the reader right up to date.

I can wholeheartedly recommend this book to any trainee in cardiology as well as those training and practising in general medicine; it provides a commonsense approach to the condition, including management based on evidence as we have it today, though recognizing that advances in the future may influence decision making. I would recommend that trainees read this book from cover to cover, and they will discover that a substantial proportion of their everyday work is no longer a mystery.

Kim Fox
Professor of Clinical Cardiology,
Royal Brompton Hospital,
London

Preface

In recent years angina pectoris, particularly unstable angina, has become an increasingly common diagnosis in patients being admitted to coronary care units (CCUs) and medical wards. A textbook written for clinicians involved in the management of patients with stable and unstable angina will fulfil a useful role. This text is aimed at physicians with an interest in cardiology, general internal medical physicians, doctors in training and staff involved in the management of patients in coronary care units and intensive care units (ICUs). It should also be of interest to primary care physicians involved in cardiovascular medicine.

This book follows a step-by-step approach to give a practical and coherent source of information. In the last decade significant advances have been made in the understanding of coronary artery pathogenesis, plaque formation and plaque instability. The role of inflammation in coronary heart disease, and the convergence of many traditional risk factors in a final common pathway leading to atherogenesis, are dealt with in some detail. It is now recognized that diabetes and obesity have become a major public health problem, and their impact on the developing plaque is discussed.

The text also outlines the approach to clinical evaluation, differential diagnosis and investigations for patients presenting with symptoms suggestive of ischaemic heart disease. There is up-to-date evidence-based information on medical strategies, interventions and surgical management. Approaches to secondary prevention and cardiac rehabilitation are described. In addition, up-to-date references for further reading are supplied. We are confident that this will be a useful text for a broad range of professionals involved in the management of patients with angina.

R.T. Murphy
E. Shelley
M.J. Walsh

Acknowledgements

We would like to acknowledge the kind assistance of a number of colleagues in the preparation and completion of this book, in particular Dr Niall Mulvihill, Dr James Meaney, Miss Marjan Jahangiri and Dr George Duffy for their help in providing images of cardiovascular medicine germane to their sub-specialty. We would like to thank all at Arnold, especially Wendy Rooke, Sarah Burrows, Jo Hargreaves, Alison Ryan, Katrina Webb and Dr Joanna Koster for their patience and cooperation at all stages of the developing project. Finally a special thanks to Ms Teresa Lawlor, for her assistance over the whole period of preparation of the book, in secretarial support and in bringing together the work of the different contributors.

Definitions and classification

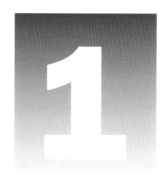

Michael J. Walsh

The definition of angina pectoris is still based on the original description supplied by Heberden,[1] in which the central feature is that of central chest pain triggered by exertion and eased by rest. It may consist of a feeling of pressure, of gripping or of aching, and if it originates in or radiates to the neck it may cause a sensation of strangulation and suffocation. It was this latter sensation which gave rise to the original term 'angina'. If the patient continues to exercise, the symptoms may become more diffuse and radiate to the arms, particularly the left arm, wrist and fingers, or to the upper abdomen or the back. Occasionally the pain occurs only in the jaw. With chronic stable angina pectoris the symptoms are invariably eased by rest. Some patients describe a 'warm-up' phenomenon with lessening of symptoms despite continuation of exercise. A common feature of angina is exacerbation by wind and lower temperatures, and patients often describe it as becoming worse if exercise is undertaken after eating.

Although the commonest cause of the symptoms of angina is ischaemic heart disease, several other conditions, such as aortic valve disease (stenosis and incompetence), hypertrophic cardiomyopathy, hypertension and anaemia, may trigger the classical symptoms in patients with normal coronary arteries.

Angina pectoris is commonly classified according to the severity of symptoms. The most commonly used classification is that of the Canadian Cardiovascular Society (see Box 1.1).

The definition of unstable angina is also currently based on the assessment of the patient's chest pain, which is said to be unstable when it increases in frequency and severity, occurs with less exertion, or may even come on at rest or when the patient is asleep, and is not as easily relieved by nitroglycerine as stable angina may be. Unstable angina will, of course, have to be differentiated from acute myocardial infarction (AMI). Braunwald[2] has described three principal presentations of unstable angina (see Box 1.2).

Box 1.1   Grading of angina pectoris by the Canadian Cardiovascular Society classification system

Class I
Ordinary physical activity, such as walking, climbing stairs, etc., does not cause angina. Angina occurs with strenuous, rapid or prolonged exertion at work or recreation.

Class II
Slight limitation of ordinary activity. Angina occurs on walking or climbing stairs rapidly, walking uphill, or walking or stair climbing after meals, or in cold, in wind, under emotional stress, or only during the first few hours after wakening. Angina occurs on walking several hundred yards on the level and climbing more than one flight of ordinary stairs at a normal pace and in normal conditions.

Class III
Marked limitation of ordinary physical activity. Angina occurs on walking one to two hundred yards on the level and climbing one flight of stairs in normal conditions and at a normal pace.

Class IV
Inability to carry on any physical activity without discomfort. Anginal symptoms may be present at rest.

Box 1.2   Classification of unstable angina according to Braunwald[2]

Class I
New-onset, severe or accelerated angina.
Patients with angina of less than 2 months duration, severe or occurring three or more times per day, or angina that is distinctly more frequent and precipitated by distinctly less exertion. No rest pain in the last 2 months.

Class II
Angina at rest. Subacute.
Patients with one or more episodes of angina at rest during the preceding month, but not within the preceding 48 h.

Class III
Angina at rest. Acute.
Patients with one or more episodes of angina at rest within the preceding 48 h.

(Continued)

Box 1.2 *(Continued)*

Clinical circumstances

Class A
Secondary unstable angina.
A clearly identified condition extrinsic to the coronary vascular bed that has intensified myocardial ischaemia (e.g. anaemia, infection, fever, hypotension, tachyarrhythmia, thyrotoxicosis, hypoxaemia secondary to respiratory failure).

Class B
Primary unstable angina.

Class C
Post-infarction unstable angina (within 2 weeks of documented myocardial infarction).

Intensity of treatment
Absence of treatment or minimal treatment.
Occurring in the presence of standard therapy for chronic stable angina (conventional doses of oral beta-blockers, nitrates and calcium antagonists).
Occurring despite maximally tolerated doses of all three above, including intravenous nitroglycerine.

References

1. Heberden W. Some account of a disorder of the breast. *Med Transactions* 1772; **2**: 59–67 (London: Royal College of Physicians).
2. Braunwald E. Unstable angina: a classification. *Circulation* 1989; **80**: 410–14.

Epidemiology of angina

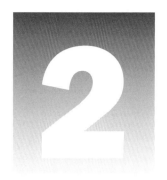

Emer Shelley

The changing epidemiology of cardiovascular disease

Any consideration of the epidemiology of angina must be set in the context of the changing patterns of morbidity and mortality from coronary heart disease (CHD). Mortality rates from CHD have declined in recent decades in many Western countries. This is probably due to a combination of reduced incidence in middle age and more effective therapies. This decrease has occurred in men and women in the UK since the mid-1980s.

The decline in the death rate may mean that there is a higher prevalence of the disease, particularly in older age groups. The age of admission with acute myocardial infarction (AMI) has increased steadily. There has been a substantial increase in the numbers of patients presenting with unstable angina, which is now a more common manifestation of acute coronary disease in some countries than is AMI.[1] Improved treatments have become available, resulting in improved survival of those admitted to hospital with an acute coronary syndrome and, overall, a longer time-course of the disease. This change in the pattern of CHD in the population has been associated with a steady increase in the prevalence of chronic heart failure, particularly among older people.

The British Regional Heart Study found that in middle age the prevalence of current angina decreased between 1978 and 1996.[2] During that time, the CHD mortality rate decreased, as did the rates of non-fatal myocardial infarction (MI), all major CHD events and first major CHD event. However, the prevalence of a history of diagnosed CHD remained unchanged. In older age groups, morbidity statistics collected by the Royal College of General Practitioners in England and Wales found that, between 1981–82 and 1991–92, the prevalence of angina pectoris increased by 63% in men and by

69% in women in the 65–74 years age group.[3,4] The corresponding increases in those aged 75 years or over were 79% and 92%, respectively.

Survey methods

In clinical practice, until recently the diagnosis of stable angina relied on obtaining a characteristic history. The prevalence in populations has frequently been estimated using a questionnaire devised by Rose and Blackburn[5] (see Box 2.1). A positive response to this questionnaire overestimates the prevalence of angina compared with a history taken by a physician.[6] The proportion of false positives is particularly high in young women.

Some population surveys have asked about a physician diagnosis of angina or AMI, some have involved a physician taking a clinical history, and some have sought electrocardiographic (ECG) evidence of ischaemia. An early report from Framingham reminded readers that estimates of the prevalence of cardiovascular disease based on survey findings are underestimates of the true prevalence: 'It should be emphasized that these prevalence rates are based on counts of survivors…who were able to attend the clinic, and the rates are, therefore, minimum estimates of true prevalence'.[7]

Surveys in general practice have utilized prescriptions for nitrates as a proxy for diagnosis of angina.[8] The prevalence figures that are obtained using prescription data provide an underestimate compared with practice-based CHD registers.

Prevalence

A substantial proportion of adults in Western populations show evidence of atherosclerotic vascular disease, which may include symptomatic CHD with

---

Box 2.1 A positive angina questionnaire[5]

1. The patient has experienced chest pain or discomfort, at the sternum or in the left anterior chest and left arm.
2. The pain occurs when walking.
3. The patient stops walking or slows down when the pain occurs.
4. Standing still relieves the symptoms.
5. Relief occurs within 10 min or less.
6. In grade 1 angina, symptoms occur when walking uphill. In grade 2 angina, symptoms also occur when walking on the level.

stable angina or a history of unstable angina or other acute coronary syndrome. Even in a country such as Spain, which has low mortality rates from CHD, the prevalence of angina as determined by the Rose Questionnaire was 7.3% in men and 7.7% in women in a national study of people aged 45 to 74 years.[9]

In countries with moderately high or high rates of atherosclerosis, the prevalence of angina increases with age in men and women. Population-based studies using a variety of research methods found that in such countries the prevalence of angina in middle age is twice as high in men as it is in women.[3] In men, the prevalence increases from 2–5% in the 45–54 years age group to 11–20% in the 65–74 years age group. In women these values are 0.5–1% and 10–14%, respectively. In the over-75s, the prevalence is similar in men and women. Based on these studies, the European Task Force estimated that in countries with high rates of atherosclerosis, 'the total prevalent number of persons with angina may be as high as 30 000–40 000 per 1 million total population'.

Overall, the prevalence of CHD declined from 1986 to 1994 in a middle-aged population sample in Northern Sweden which was part of the Swedish MONICA Project (Multinational Monitoring of Trends and Cardiovascular Disease).[10] The percentage with a history of AMI decreased from 4.6% to 2.0%. The prevalence of angina in women declined from 6% to 3%. However, the prevalence in men remained unchanged at 3%.

Given the changing epidemiology of cardiovascular disease and the ageing of the population in developed countries, the prevalence of stable angina in older people in the community is of particular interest. A cohort study in three communities in the USA included over 8000 men and women aged 65 years or older.[11] The prevalence of angina, as determined by the Rose Questionnaire, across the communities was in the range 3–4% in men and 4–6% in women. The prevalence of angina was higher when individuals with chest pain on exertion which did not meet the Rose Questionnaire criteria were included in the definition (5–7% in men and 7–9% in women). Those with chest pain on exertion had a significantly increased risk of CHD death, which was independent of other risk factors for CHD.

A population-based study of people aged 64–97 years in rural Finland found a prevalence of stable angina of 9% in men and 5% in women.[12] However, the total prevalence of CHD was much higher when a documented history of a cardiovascular disease and ECG findings were taken into account, at 37.7% (range 33.4–42.0%) in men and 42.0% (range 38.3–45.6%) in women.

The very high prevalence of chronic vascular disease in older people in the UK was demonstrated by a study which assessed the presence of femoral atherosclerosis using ultrasound.[13] Nearly two-thirds (64%) of the random sample of 784 subjects showed evidence of femoral plaque. The prevalence was higher in men (67%) than in women (59%), and femoral plaque was more common in those with previous ischaemic heart disease or angina. The risk was significantly increased in those who were current or ex-smokers, with raised serum total cholesterol and plasma fibrinogen levels. Frequent exercise and a high level of high-density-lipoprotein cholesterol (HDL-cholesterol) were associated with lower risk of femoral plaque.

The Health Survey for England 1991 showed the typical pattern of an increase in angina-type symptoms with age.[14] The higher prevalence of such symptoms in women under 50 years of age compared with men has been found in other surveys, but has not been associated with ECG abnormalities or excess mortality.

The Medical Research Council Cognitive Function and Ageing Study (CFAS) was carried out using random population samples in three urban and two rural locations in England and Wales.[15] From the initial interviews conducted between 1989 and 1994, it was estimated that nearly 7% of men and 5% of women in the 65–74 years age group had been diagnosed as having angina but had no history of heart attack or stroke. The corresponding prevalences for those aged 75 years or over were 7% and 8% (see Table 2.1). Almost half of those surveyed either had angina, heart attack or stroke, or had a condition which put them at high risk of developing symptomatic cardiovascular disease.

The findings of the CFAS were compared with those of the Health Survey for England 1992.[15,16] The latter only included people living in private households, whereas the CFAS included those in residential accommodation

Table 2.1
The prevalence of cardiovascular disease and related conditions in men and women in the MRC Cognitive Function and Ageing Study (CFAS) and in the *Health Survey for England 1992*[15,16]

Condition	CFAS		Health Survey for England 1992	
Age (years)	65–74	≥75	65–74	≥75
Heart attack or stroke				
Men	19.3	22.3	15	16
Women	9.9	15.6	8	12
Angina but not heart attack or stroke				
Men	6.6	6.9	6	11
Women	5.4	7.9	6	6
Only hypertension or diabetes				
Men	22.1	18.6	24	19
Women	29.4	25.1	30	25
None of the above				
Men	52.1	52.1	56	54
Women	55.3	52.4	56	57

who were registered with a general practitioner. As would be expected, the prevalence was higher when those in residential homes were included.

Incidence

In the 20-year follow-up of the Framingham Study cohort, the annual incidence of angina pectoris in men was found to be 0.3% in the 45–54 years age group, 0.8% in the 55–64 years age group and 0.6% in the 65–74 years age group.[7] The corresponding incidence figures in women were 0.2%, 0.6% and 0.6%, respectively. A lower proportion of coronary disease presented as angina in men than in women. However, the overall incidence of coronary disease was higher in men than in women, and hence the incidence of angina was higher in men up to the age of 65 years.

The lifetime risk of developing CHD (angina pectoris, coronary insufficiency, MI or death from CHD) was estimated for participants in the Framingham Heart Study.[17] The risk at age 40 years was 48.6% for men and 31.7% for women. At age 70 years, the lifetime risk was 34.9% for men and 24.2% for women. Only a small proportion of those who developed CHD had isolated angina pectoris, with most patients developing other manifestations of the disease.

The Seven Countries Study of men aged 40–59 years at baseline in the late 1950s and early 1960s found an annual incidence of angina of 0.1% in Japan, Greece and Croatia, 0.2–0.4% in Italy, Serbia, The Netherlands and the USA, and 0.6–1.1% in Finland.[18]

Based on a study of referrals by general practitioners to a chest pain clinic, it was estimated that there are 22 600 new cases of angina each year in the UK.[19]

Changes over time in new (incident) cases of ischaemic heart disease presenting to general practice were examined in five practices (with a total population of nearly 40 000 patients) in the Trent Region of England.[20] A retrospective analysis of cases presenting between 1993 and 1997 found that just over half (54.0%) of new cases were diagnosed as having angina pectoris, 26.9% as having an AMI, 18.8% as having ischaemic heart disease and 0.3% as having coronary atherosclerosis. The incidence was highest in January and on Mondays and Fridays. There was a downward trend in the total number of new cases over the 5-year period, with an increase in the proportion of cases presenting with AMI.

Risk factors

There is a large measure of agreement internationally with regard to the factors which increase the risk of CHD, including angina. A World Health

Organization (WHO) Expert Committee which reported in 1982 stated that 'the major determinants of population rates of CHD had now been identified: an inappropriate national diet aggravated by physical inactivity and overweight (reflected in the mass raising of blood lipids and blood pressure), and widespread cigarette-smoking'.[21] Smoking, raised blood pressure and raised blood cholesterol levels may be regarded as the three 'classic' risk factors for CHD.

The Joint European Task Force on Prevention of Coronary Heart Disease in Clinical Practice has categorized the main factors which alter risk into personal characteristics which are not modifiable (such as age and sex), and lifestyle factors and biochemical or physiological characteristics which may be amenable to change (see Table 2.2).[22]

The British Regional Heart Study (see Box 2.2) followed a cohort of 7735 men aged 40–59 years at baseline, chosen from general practices in 24 UK towns for three successive 5-year periods.[23] For men with no recall of a diagnosis of CHD, the established risk factors, namely serum total cholesterol, HDL cholesterol, systolic and diastolic blood pressure, physical activity, body mass index (BMI), alcohol intake, diabetes mellitus, parental history and evidence of CHD on chest pain questionnaire or on ECG, were predictive of CHD events occurring in each of the 5-year follow-up periods.

Follow-up confirmed the North–South gradient in CHD incidence in the UK, with higher rates in towns in Scotland and Northern England compared with Southern England, ranging from 1.07% to 0.52% per annum

Table 2.2
Lifestyles and other characteristics associated with increased risk of future CHD[22]

Personal characteristics (non-modifiable)	Lifestyles	Biochemical or physiological characteristics (modifiable)
Age	Diet high in saturated fat, cholesterol and calories	Elevated blood pressure
Sex	Tobacco smoking	Elevated plasma total cholesterol (LDL-cholesterol)
Family history of CHD or other atherosclerotic vascular disease at early age (in men < 55 years, in women < 65 years)	Excess alcohol consumption	Low plasma HDL-cholesterol
Personal history of CHD or other atherosclerotic vascular disease	Physical inactivity	Elevated plasma triglycerides
		Hyperglycaemia/diabetes Obesity Thrombogenic factors

during 15 years of follow-up.[24] Much of the variation was accounted for by established risk variables, with occupational social class and height being included in the model. Similar associations between the traditional risk factors and risk of CHD were found in the West of Scotland Coronary Prevention Study.[25]

Box 2.2   Some results from the British Regional Heart Study

A baseline survey during 1978–80 of 7735 men aged 40 to 59 years chosen randomly from 24 general practices in England, Wales and Scotland found that 25% of the men showed evidence of CHD.[42] On questionnaire, 14% of the men had possible MI with or without angina. ECG evidence was present in nearly 15% of the men, of either MI (4%) or myocardial ischaemia (10%). ECG evidence of a past AMI increased fourfold across the age range. There was considerable overlap between the groups with positive question-naires and those with positive ECGs. Nevertheless, about half of those with possible MI combined with angina on questionnaire had no evidence of ischaemia on resting ECG, and half of those with definite MI on ECG had no history of chest pain.

The relative risk associated with a diagnosis of CHD at baseline declined substantially over time.[43] Comparison of outcome in those with evidence of disease at baseline (preva-lent disease) compared with those who were newly diagnosed (incident cases) demon-strated the better prognosis of men surviving the initial years after the event. Risk of death or of a cardiovascular event (major CHD event, total and cardiovascular mortality, stroke or major cardiovascular event) increased strongly from those with no evidence of CHD through increasing levels of symptomatic or diagnosed disease. For all cardiovascular outcomes other than stroke, diagnosed MI was associated with a much poorer prognosis compared with those with diagnosed or symptomatic angina. When adjusted to an average age of 50 years, the proportion of men who survived for 15 years free of a new major cardiovascular event was 44% for diagnosed MI, 66% for diagnosed angina, 68% for angina symptoms and 79% for those with no ischaemic heart disease.

Exertional chest pain was a strong indicator of major coronary risk. Persistent symptoms were associated with severe disease and a poor prognosis compared with those men in whom the symptoms varied over time.[44]

Alcohol, smoking and risk of death

When the men with a physician diagnosis of CHD were followed for nearly 13 years, ex-drinkers were found to have the highest risk of death from CHD, all cardiovascular diseases or all causes. There were no differences in the risk of death between occasional drinkers and lifelong non-drinkers or light drinkers. Moderate or heavy drinkers had increased risks of death compared with occasional drinkers. The excess risk of death was confined to men with a history of acute MI, not to those with a history of angina without an acute MI. Stopping smoking during the first 5 years of follow-up was associated with a substantial reduction in the risk of death from cardiovascular diseases and from all causes compared with those who continued to smoke.

(Continued)

Box 2.2 *(Continued)*

The metabolic syndrome

The associations between hypertension, hyperglycaemia, lipid and other metabolic abnormalities were examined in a subgroup of men who had no history of CHD, diabetes or stroke, and who were living in 18 of the towns.[45] The 'full metabolic syndrome' of hypertension, hyperglycaemia and dyslipidaemia was found in 3% of the men. Men with hypertension had significantly higher levels of total cholesterol, triglycerides, blood glucose and urate, and showed more clustering of hyperglycaemia and dyslipidaemia, compared with normotensives.

Physical activity

In 1992, 12 to 14 years after the baseline study, the men were reassessed and followed for a further 5 years.[46] Among those with diagnosed CHD in 1992, the lowest risk (after adjustment for potential confounders) during follow-up for all causes and for cardiovascular mortality was seen in the light physical activity group (relative risk 0.42; 95% confidence intervals 0.52, 0.71) and moderate physical activity group (relative risk 0.47; 95% confidence intervals 0.24, 0.92) compared with those who were inactive or only occasionally active. The reduced risk associated with light or moderate physical activity was seen in men with diagnosed heart disease both under and over the age of 65 years. These levels of activity were also found to benefit the men who experienced chest pain or severe breathlessness on exertion, as well as those who were asymptomatic on exertion. Men who were inactive at baseline but who had started at least light activity by the 1992 follow-up, despite the diagnosis of heart disease, also showed lower mortality rates than those who remained sedentary throughout (relative risk 0.58; 95% confidence intervals 0.33, 1.03; $P = 0.06$).

Overall, the men with diagnosed heart disease who were involved in recreational activities for 4 or more hours at weekends had a significantly lower risk (after adjustment) of all-cause and cardiovascular mortality compared with those who were not this active. There were also significant reductions in mortality in men who walked for more than 40 min per day, and in those who engaged in moderate or strenuous gardening.

Physical activity and diabetes

In men who were free of CHD, stroke or diabetes at baseline there were significant trend relationships after 17 years (after adjustment for a range of potential confounders) between level of physical activity and factors associated with risk of cardiovascular disease or diabetes, including diastolic blood pressure, HDL-cholesterol, triglycerides, serum insulin and urate levels.[47] The risk of developing CHD was reduced in those men who were active at the time of the initial survey. The lowest risk of heart disease occurred in those who were moderately active, and no additional benefit was obtained from taking more vigorous exercise. The risk of developing diabetes was inversely related to the level of activity reported at baseline. There was evidence that the favourable influence of physical activity on the risk of diabetes was mediated through components of the insulin resistance syndrome.

There is evidence of clustering of metabolically linked risk factors, including low HDL-cholesterol levels and raised BMI, systolic blood pressure, triglycerides, glucose and serum total cholesterol.[26] Weight gain (2.25 kg, 5 pounds) was associated with an increase in the sum of these risk factors, and the converse was true for weight loss. Clustering of risk factors was associated with a greatly increased risk of CHD in both men and women.

It is now recognized that a diet which is high in energy and saturated fats and low in unsaturated fats and antioxidants is associated with increased risk of atherosclerotic vascular disease.[22] Attention to diet is an important component of secondary prevention (see Chapter 12, p. 184).

The relationship between alcohol intake and risk of CHD is complex. Identified alcoholics and problem drinkers have an increased risk of CHD, reflecting the association between alcohol intake and raised blood pressure and abnormal triglyceride metabolism.[27] Studies in several countries have shown that those with moderate alcohol intake have a lower CHD risk than abstainers. There are plausible mechanisms for such a protective effect of alcohol, including its association with higher HDL-cholesterol levels, and the antioxidant effects of wine.

Trends in risk factors for cardiovascular disease in England were studied by comparing the findings in men aged 20–64 years in the 1984 Health and Lifestyle Survey 'first sweep' and those in the 1993 Health Survey for England.[28] In parallel with the decline in cardiovascular disease death rates, the prevalence of risk factors decreased. Most of these changes appeared to occur equally across the spectrum of social classes. There was a non-significant increase in the relative risk of angina among the less well off from 1.75 in 1984 to 1.96 in 1993. The authors concluded that the changes in risk factors as measured in the surveys did not explain the pattern of widening inequality in cardiovascular mortality.

The increasing prevalence of diabetes is a cause for concern. Telephone surveys in the USA found that the prevalence of self-reported diabetes increased from 4.9% of adults in 1990 to 6.5% in 1998.[29] The prevalence was strongly correlated with the prevalence of obesity. The increase occurred in men and women, and across the spectrum of age, ethnic groups and education levels. It occurred in most of the states included in the Behavioural Risk Factor Surveillance Survey, but the extent of the increase varied across states.

Haemostatic factors have been shown to be associated with an increased risk of CHD.[30] It was concluded from the Edinburgh Artery Study that increased coagulation activity with raised plasma fibrinogen levels and disturbed fibrinolysis are predictors of future vascular events, including ischaemic heart disease and stroke. Subjects with angina pectoris who developed a thrombotic vascular event also showed evidence of leucocyte activation, with raised tissue plasminogen activator and leucocyte elastase levels.[31] Blood viscosity, haematocrit and white-cell count were independent predictors of incident CHD in the West of Scotland Coronary Prevention Study, while fibrinogen predicted risk of mortality.[32]

The role of infections and inflammation in the aetiology of CHD is under investigation. High levels of antibody to *Chlamydia pneumoniae* (*Cp*) were found in the Helsinki Heart Study in CHD cases compared with controls.[33] *Cp* is a common cause of respiratory infection, is vasotropic and is frequently found in human atheromatous lesions.[34] However, the extent to which *Cp* or other infectious agents play a causal role in atherosclerosis or are involved in ongoing inflammation, exacerbating acute and chronic atherosclerotic processes, remains unclear.

Elevated homocysteine levels are associated with an increased risk of thrombosis in patients who present with acute coronary syndromes.[35] Furthermore, the extent of myocardial damage in such patients has been correlated with the plasma homocysteine concentration on admission.

In addition to lifestyle and genetic factors, environmental factors (including the social, cultural and occupational milieu, and even prenatal factors) have been shown to influence the risk of CHD. The effect of prenatal exposure to maternal malnutrition on the development of CHD was studied in a small sample of people born around the time of the Dutch famine in 1944–45.[36] The prevalence of CHD was higher among those who were exposed to malnutrition during early gestation compared with those who were not exposed in this way. People with CHD tended to have lower birth weights and smaller head circumferences. The effect of maternal malnutrition was not evident in those exposed in mid or late gestation, and was independent of birth weight.

The association between low birth weight in relation to the duration of gestation and increased risk of CHD, stroke, hypertension and non-insulin-dependent diabetes has been replicated in studies in a number of countries.[37] It is postulated that the associations are the consequences of 'programming', whereby a stimulus at a critical time in early life has permanent effects on structure, physiology and metabolism. There is evidence that maternal body composition and dietary balance during pregnancy may affect fetal development and alter the risk of CHD in later life.

Some of the differences in incidence between social groups can be attributed to lifestyle and behavioural factors. The Whitehall Study of civil servants found that the risk of CHD death was inversely associated with employment grade.[38] The main risk factors, including glucose intolerance and diabetes, could only explain one-third of the gradient.[39] Comparing the older retired group with the younger pre-retirement group, the differentials in mortality remained, but were less pronounced.

In the Whitehall Study, employment grade was strongly related to father's social class.[40] However, adult socio-economic status was a more important predictor of CHD morbidity than was social status earlier in life. Evidence from the 1993 Health Survey for England found that men in 'high-strain' jobs (i.e. high demand and low control) were at increased risk of angina and possible MI, as measured by the Rose Questionnaire.[41] Although some of the unexplained differences between social classes may reflect the inadequacies of the risk assessment and adjustment processes, there is strong evidence that social and cultural factors from childhood onwards influence the risk of developing CHD in adulthood.

Natural history and prognosis

Patient and disease characteristics were studied in a non-hospitalized population of 5125 patients with a diagnosis of stable angina who were attending a total of 1266 primary care physicians in the USA.[48] The mean age of the group was 69 years, 53% were women, and 70% had more than one associated illness. The median frequency of angina was approximately two episodes per week. Effort angina was present in 90% of patients, 47% also had rest angina and 34% had angina precipitated by mental stress.

Follow-up over a 7-year period of patients being treated with nitrates for ischaemic heart disease found that 26% were admitted urgently with chest pain and 15% were referred to the medical outpatient department. Overall, the death rate was 6% per annum.[49]

Follow-up in Rochester, Minnesota, of residents first diagnosed as having coronary artery disease during the 1960s or 1970s showed that women with angina pectoris as an initial diagnosis, but not those with MI, had a longer survival and lower risk of subsequent infarction or sudden death compared with men of a similar age.[50]

The Framingham Heart Study also found that women had a more favourable prognosis than men after the onset of angina.[51] Follow-up of the Framingham Study population also found that the overall risk of developing congestive heart failure was 20% in both men and women.[52] Hypertension was the most important modifiable risk factor for the development of heart failure, indicating overlap with the group at increased risk of angina.

A subgroup of patients presents with chest pain similar to angina but with normal coronary arteries on angiography. Follow-up of a group of such men of mean age 48 years found an incidence of MI of less than 1% per annum.[53] These men were more likely to have classical risk factors for coronary artery disease. There was also a low incidence of more severe angina with the emergence of coronary artery pathology.

No significant differences were found when atherogenic, haemostatic, inflammatory and some genetic variables were compared in patients with a previous uncomplicated AMI and patients with long-standing stable angina.[54] This suggests that acute coronary events occur as random events against a background of atherosclerosis. Nowadays, the pattern of disease is affected by therapies which alter the natural history and improve the prognosis.

Unstable angina

The diagnosis of unstable angina or non-ST-segment elevation MI constitutes the largest proportion of admissions to coronary care units.[1] The risk of an ischaemic event during the acute phase and the following 3 months is nearly 50%. In patients with stable angina, stenoses associated with previous episodes of unstable angina are more likely to progress than those that are not associated with unstable angina.[55] It is postulated that unstable atherosclerotic plaques, even those which have been stable for more than 3 months, may retain the potential for rapid progression to total occlusion. Risk stratification enables hospitalization of those patients who are at highest risk.[1]

A risk score for developing at least one of the primary end-points (death, new or recurrent MI, or severe ischaemia requiring urgent revascularization) was derived from the outcomes of the Thrombolysis in Myocardial Infarction (TIMI IIB) trial and the ESSENCE trial.[56] The seven TIMI risk score predictor variables were age 65 years or older, at least three risk factors for CHD, prior coronary stenosis of 50% or more, ST-segment deviation on ECG at presentation, at least two anginal events in the previous 24 h, use of aspirin during the previous 7 days, and elevated serum cardiac markers. Event rates increased significantly as the TIMI risk score increased in the TIMI IIB cohort, from just under 5% for a score of 0 or 1, to 20% with a score of 4, to 41% in those who scored 6 or 7. This pattern was confirmed in the three validation groups. The slope of the increase in event rates was significantly lower in those treated with enoxaparin (a low-molecular-weight heparin). The TIMI risk score appears to be of value in categorizing a patient's risk of death or ischaemic event, and it provides a basis for clinical decision-making.

A series of patients with unstable angina was followed for a mean period of just over 3 years in the FRISC study in Sweden.[57] Predictors of both short-term and longer-term risk of death from cardiac causes included the level of troponin T (a marker of myocardial damage) and C-reactive protein (a marker of inflammation) at the time of presentation.[57] Around 30–40% of patients with unstable angina have elevated levels of serum troponin T and/or I, often with normal creatine kinase-MB levels.[1] These patients have a 5-fold to 15-fold increase in the risk of a future cardiac ischaemic event.

Plasma levels of secretory non-pancreatic type II phospholipase A2 (sPLA2) are increased in a number of chronic inflammatory diseases.[58] Japanese patients with unstable angina have been found to have higher levels of sPLA2 than either patients with stable angina or control subjects. Furthermore, those unstable angina patients with the highest levels of sPLA2 had a significantly higher probability of developing clinical coronary events in the next 2 years, independent of other risk factors, including C-reactive protein.

Myocardial infarction

In one series, 25% of patients who presented with an MI had prodromal angina during the 24 h before the MI.[59] Such patients were more likely to have a patent infarct-related vessel than were those without prodromal angina. In-hospital mortality and 5-year survival rates were better in those who experienced prodromal angina. In contrast, there was no difference in mortality between patients with angina at any time in the past (58% of patients) and those without such a history. Better outcomes in patients with prodromal angina have been found in other studies, associated with smaller infarct size and better left ventricular function.[60] Preconditioning has been demonstrated in animal models, where an earlier episode of ischaemia results in better tolerance of a later, more prolonged episode. Higher canalization rates following thrombolysis have been demonstrated in patients with prodromal angina compared with those without antecedent angina.

In Irish men under the age of 60 years who had an MI between the mid-1960s and the mid-1970s, 24% of survivors had angina pectoris during the year after the infarct.[61] The proportion who reported angina increased to 30%, 30% and 44% after 5, 10 and 15 years, respectively. Mortality during periods in which patients reported angina was higher than that in symptom-free periods.

Patients with a history of angina and those with diabetes were more likely to present late for treatment of AMI in a large series of Medicare beneficiaries in the USA.[62] Other factors associated with presentation more than 6 h after the onset of symptoms included initial evaluation as an outpatient, daytime presentation, and being female, black or of low socio-economic status. These findings have implications for the education of patients with angina with regard to the symptoms of an AMI, and the advised actions in such circumstances.

After coronary artery bypass surgery

In the Coronary Artery Surgery Study (CASS) registry, 24% of patients had recurrence of angina in the first year after surgery, and 40% had recurrence after 6 years.[63] These patients were at increased risk of both MI and reoperation. Predictors of recurrence of angina after surgery included preoperative angina, use of vein grafts only, previous MI, incomplete revascularization, female gender, smoking and younger age.

Outcome in men and women was compared in a series of patients who had undergone coronary artery bypass surgery in Ontario, Canada.[64] Female patients were older, but some potential indicators of poor outcome (e.g. ejection fraction less than 35%) were more frequent in the male patients. After adjustment for other risk variables, female gender was not an independent predictor of early mortality, but there was a weak association with perioperative complications. Recurrent angina was more frequent in women. However, survival after 5 years was higher in women (93.1%) than in men (90.0%), and after adjustment for other risk variables, female gender was protective for late survival (risk ratio 0.40; 95% confidence interval 0.16–0.74; $P < 0.005$).

After angioplasty

The RITA trial[65] compared the outcome in patients with angina who were randomized to either coronary bypass surgery or angioplasty. After 2 years, 31% of patients in the angioplasty group had angina, compared with 22% in the surgical group. However, the recurrence of severe angina was similar in both groups.

In the RITA trial, there was a close relationship at baseline between the grade of angina and measures of quality of life (energy levels, pain, emotional difficulties, sleep, social isolation and mobility).[66] Surgery and angioplasty resulted in similar improvements in quality of life and return to employment during the 3 years after the intervention.

Outcome after stenting for coronary artery disease outside the emergency setting was compared in a series of 1001 women and 3263 men in two tertiary referral centres in Germany.[67] The women were significantly older (mean age 69 vs. 63 years) and were more likely to have diabetes, hypertension or hypercholesterolaemia. However, despite these differences, the women had less extensive coronary artery disease, were less likely to have a history of MI, and had better left ventricular function than the men. The frequency of death or non-fatal MI was higher in the women (3.1%) than in the men (1.8%) during the first 30 days after stenting. However, at 1 year the outcome was similar for women (combined event rate 6.0%) and men (5.8%). The strongest prognostic factors were diabetes in women and age in men.

Secondary prevention

Patients with established CHD are in the highest-priority category for prevention activities in clinical practice.[22] The overall objective in patients with stable angina is to reduce the progression of atherosclerotic coronary artery disease and the risk of fatal thrombosis, and thereby to decrease the risk of a non-fatal or fatal coronary event. Specific objectives of secondary prevention in patients with angina are to modify the patient's risk factors, to use pro-phylactic drugs and to screen the patient's closest relatives. With the advent of improved treatments, including cholesterol-lowering agents, it is likely that the prognosis for patients with angina is better now than at any time in the past. Secondary prevention and cardiac rehabilitation are described in Chapter 12 (p. 177).

Summary

The European Task Force on Angina Pectoris estimated that, in countries with high rates of CHD, the prevalence of angina is approximately 30 000 to 40 000 per 1 million members of the population. Despite an increase in the age of onset in many developed countries, the prevalence of angina is rising because of a longer time-course of the disease and the availability of more effective treatments. The disease is usually slowly progressive. Women with angina have a longer survival and lower risk of subsequent infarction or sudden death than men of a similar age. Although angina is a serious condition, the symptoms and prognosis can be substantially improved both by treatment and by preventive measures to address the patient's risk factors for coronary heart disease.

References

1. Théroux P, Willerson JT, Armstrong PW. Progress in the treatment of acute coronary syndromes: a 50-year perspective. *Circulation* 2000; **102 (Supplement 4)**: IV2–13.
2. Lampe FC, Morris RW, Whincup PH, Walker M, Ebrahim S, Shaper AG. Is the prevalence of coronary heart disease falling in British men? *Heart* 2001; **86**: 499–505.
3. Julian DG, Bertrand ME, Hjalmarson A *et al.* Management of stable angina pectoris. Recommendations of the Task Force of the European Society of Cardiology. *Eur Heart J* 1997; **18**: 394–413.
4. British Heart Foundation. *Coronary heart disease statistics.* London: British Heart Foundation, 1994.
5. Rose GA, Blackburn H. *Cardiovascular survey methods.* Geneva: World Health Organization, 1968.
6. Hagman M, Johsson D, Wilhelmsen L. Prevalence of angina pectoris and myocardial infarction in a general population sample of Swedish men. *Acta Med Scand* 1977; **201**: 571–7.

7. Dawber TE, Moore FE, Mann GV. Measuring the risk of coronary heart disease in adult population groups. A symposium: coronary heart disease in the Framingham Study. *Am J Pub Health* 1957; **47**: 4–23.

8. Bottomley A. Methodology for assessing the prevalence of angina in primary care using practice-based information in northern England. *J Epidemiol Commun Health* 1997; **51**: 87–9.

9. Cosin J, Asin E, Marrugat J *et al.* Prevalence of angina pectoris in Spain. PANES study group. *Eur J Epidemiol* 1999; **15**: 323–30.

10. Glader EL, Stegmayr B. Declining prevalence of angina pectoris in middle-aged men and women. A population-based study within the Northern Sweden MONICA Project. Multinational monitoring of trends and cardiovascular disease. *J Intern Med* 1999; **246**: 285–91.

11. LaCroix AZ, Guralnik JM, Curb D, Wallace RB, Ostfeld AM, Hennekens CH. Chest pain and coronary heart disease mortality among older men and women in three communities. *Circulation* 1990; **81**: 437–46.

12. Ahto M, Isoaho R, Puolijoke H *et al.* Prevalence of coronary heart disease, associated manifestations and electrocardiographic findings in elderly Finns. *Age Ageing* 1998; **27**: 729–37.

13. Leng GC, Papacosta O, Whincup P *et al.* Femoral atherosclerosis in an older British population: prevalence and risk factors. *Atherosclerosis* 2000; **152**: 167–74.

14. Office of Population Censuses and Surveys. *Health Survey for England 1991.* London: HMSO, 1993.

15. Parker CJ, Morgan K, Dewey ME and the Analysis Group of the MRC Cognitive Function and Ageing Study. Physical illness and disability among elderly people in England and Wales: the Medical Research Council Cognitive Function and Ageing Study. *J Epidemiol Commun Health* 1997; **51**: 494–501.

16. Office of Population Censuses and Surveys. *Health Survey for England 1992.* London: HMSO, 1994.

17. Lloyd-Jones DM, Larson MG, Beiser A, Levy D. Lifetime risk of developing coronary heart disease. *Lancet* 1999; **353**: 89–92.

18. Keys A. *Seven countries: a multivariate analysis of death and coronary heart disease.* Cambridge, MA: Harvard University Press, 1980.

19. Gandhi MM, Lampe FC, Wood DA. Incidence, clinical characteristics and short-term prognosis of angina pectoris. *Br Heart J* 1995; **73**: 193–8.

20. Meal AG, Pringle M, Hammersley V. Time changes in new cases of ischaemic heart disease in general practice. *Fam Pract* 2000; **17**: 394–400.

21. World Health Organization Expert Committee. *Prevention of coronary heart disease.* Technical Report Series 678. Geneva: World Health Organization, 1982.

22. Wood D, De Backer G, Faergeman O, Graham I, Mancia G, Pyorala K. Prevention of coronary heart disease in clinical practice. Recommendations of the Second Joint Task Force of European and other Societies on Coronary Prevention. *Eur Heart J* 1998; **19**: 1434–503.

23. Wannamethee SG, Shaper AG, Whincup PH, Walker M. Role of risk factors for major coronary heart disease events with increasing length of follow-up. *Heart* 1999; **81**: 374–9.

24. Morris RW, Whincup PH, Lampe FC, Walker M, Wannamethee SG, Shaper AG. Geographic variation in incidence of coronary heart disease in Britain: the contribution of established risk factors. *Heart* 2001; **86**: 277–83.

25. West of Scotland Coronary Prevention Study Group. Baseline risk factors and their association with outcome in the West of Scotland Coronary Prevention Study. *Am J Cardiol* 1997; **79**: 756–62.

26. Wilson PW, Kannel WB, Silbershatz H, D'Agostino RB. Clustering of metabolic factors and coronary heart disease. *Arch Intern Med* 1999; **159**: 1104–9.

27. Marmot MG. Alcohol and coronary heart disease. *Int J Epidemiol* 2001; **30**: 724–9.

28. Bartley M, Fitzpatrick R, Firth D, Marmot M. Social distribution of cardiovascular risk factors: change among men in England 1984–1993. *J Epidemiol Commun Health* 2000; **54**: 806–14.

29. Mokdad AH, Ford ES, Bowman BA *et al.* Diabetes trends in the US: 1990–1998. *Diabetes Care* 2000; **23**: 1278–83.

30. Smith FB, Lee AJ, Fowkes FG, Price JF, Rumley A, Lowe GD. Haemostatic factors as predictors of ischaemic heart disease and stroke in the Edinburgh Artery Study. *Arterioscler Thromb Vasc Biol* 1999; **19**: 493–8.

31. Smith FB, Fowkes FG, Rumley A, Lee AJ, Lowe GD, Hau CM. Tissue plasminogen activator and leucocyte elastase as predictors of cardiovascular events in subjects with angina pectoris: Edinburgh Artery Study. *Eur Heart J* 2000; **21**: 1607–13.

32. Lowe G, Rumley A, Norrie J *et al.* Blood rheology, cardiovascular risk factors and cardiovascular disease: the West of Scotland Coronary Prevention Study. *Thromb Haemost* 2000; **84**: 553–8.

33. Roivainen M, Viik-Kajander M, Palosuo T *et al.* Infections, inflammation, and the risk of coronary heart disease. *Circulation* 2000; **101**: 252–7.

34. Anderson JL, Muhlestein JB. The ACADEMIC study in perspective (Azithromycin in Coronary Artery Disease: Elimination of Myocardial Infection with *Chlamydia*). *J Infect Dis* 2000: **181 (Supplement 3)**: S569–71.

35. Al-Obaidi MK, Stubbs PJ, Collinson P, Conroy R, Graham I, Noble MI. Elevated homocysteine levels are associated with increased ischemic

myocardial injury in acute coronary syndromes. *J Am Coll Cardiol* 2000; **36**: 1217–22.

36. Roseboom TJ, van der Meulen JH, Osmond C *et al.* Coronary heart disease after prenatal exposure to the Dutch famine, 1944–45. *Heart* 2000; **84**: 595–8.

37. Godfrey KM, Barker DJ. Fetal programming and adult health. *Pub Health Nutr* 2001; **4**: 611–24.

38. Hemingway H, Shipley M, Macfarlane P, Marmot M. Impact of socio-economic status on coronary mortality in people with symptoms, electro-graphic abnormalities, both or neither: the original Whitehall Study 25-year follow-up. *J Epidemiol Commun Health* 2000; **54**: 510–16.

39. Van Rossum CT, Shipley MJ, van de Mheen H, Grobee DE, Marmot MG. Employment grade differences in cause-specific mortality. A 25-year follow-up of civil servants from the first Whitehall Study. *J Epidemiol Commun Health* 2000; **54**: 178–84.

40. Marmot M, Shipley M, Brunner E, Hemingway H. Relative contribution of early life and adult socioeconomic factors to adult morbidity in the Whitehall II Study. *J Epidemiol Commun Health* 2001; **55**: 301–7.

41. Sacker A, Bartley MJ, Frith D, Fitzpatrick RM, Marmot MG. The relationship between job strain and coronary heart disease: evidence from an English sample of the working male population. *Psychol Med* 2001; **31**: 279–90.

42. Shaper AG, Cook DG, Walker M, Macfarlane PW. Prevalence of ischaemic heart disease in middle-aged British men. *Br Heart J* 1984; **51**: 595–605.

43. Lampe FC, Whincup PH, Wannamethee SG, Shaper AG, Walker M, Ebrahim S. The natural history of prevalent ischaemic heart disease in middle-aged men. *Eur Heart J* 2000; **13**: 1052–62.

44. Lampe FC, Whincup PH, Shaper AG, Wannamethee SG, Walker M, Ebrahim S. Variability of angina symptoms and the risk of major ischemic heart disease events. *Am J Epidemiol* 2001; **153**: 1173–82.

45. Wannamethee SG, Shaper AG, Durrington PN, Perry IJ. Hypertension, serum insulin, obesity and the metabolic syndrome. *J Hum Hypertens* 1998; **12**: 735–41.

46. Wannamethee SG, Shaper AG, Walker M. Physical activity and mortality in older men with diagnosed coronary heart disease. *Circulation* 2000; **102**: 1358–63.

47. Wannamethee SG, Shaper AG, Alberti KG. Physical activity, metabolic factors, and the incidence of coronary heart disease and type 2 diabetes. *Arch Intern Med* 2000; **160**: 2108–16.

48. Pepine CJ. Angina pectoris in a contemporary population: characteristics and therapeutic implications. TIDES investigators. *Cardiovasc Drugs Ther* 1998; **12 (Supplement 3)**: 211–16.

49. Clarke KW, Gray D, Hampton JR. Implication of prescriptions for nitrates: 7-year follow-up of patients treated for angina in general practice. *Br Heart J* 1994; **72**: 38–40.

50. Orencia A, Bailey K, Yawn BP, Kottke TE. Effect of gender on long-term outcome of angina pectoris and myocardial infarction/sudden unexpected death. *J Am Med Assoc* 1993; **269**: 2392–7.

51. Murabito JM, Evans JC, Larson MG, Levy D. Endothelial function/coronary blood flow/coronary disease syndromes. Prognosis after onset of coronary heart disease: an investigation of differences in outcome between the sexes according to initial coronary disease presentation. *Circulation* 1993; **88**: 2548–55.

52. Lloyd-Jones DM. The risk of congestive heart failure: sobering lessons from the Framingham Heart Study. *Curr Cardiol Rep* 2001; **3**: 184–90.

53. Lichtlen PR, Bargheer K, Wenzlaff P. Long-term prognosis of patients with angina-like chest pain and normal coronary angiographic findings. *J Am Coll Cardiol* 1995; **25**: 1013–18.

54. Bogaty P, Robitaille NM, Solymoss S *et al.* Atherogenic, hemostatic, and other potential risk markers in subjects with previous isolated myocardial infarction compared with long-standing uncomplicated stable angina. *Am Heart J* 1998; **136**: 884–93.

55. Kaski JC, Chen L, Crook R, Cox I, Tousoulis D, Chester MR. Coronary stenosis progression differs in patients with stable angina pectoris with and without a previous history of unstable angina. *Eur Heart J* 1996; **17**: 1488–94.

56. Antman EM, Cohen M, Bernink PJ *et al.* The TIMI risk score for unstable angina/non-ST elevation MI: a method for prognostication and therapeutic decision making. *J Am Med Assoc* 2000; **284**: 835–42.

57. Lindahl B, Toss H, Siegbahn A, Venge P, Wallentin L for the FRISC Study Group. Markers of myocardial damage and inflammation in relation to long-term mortality in unstable coronary artery disease. *N Engl J Med* 2000; **343**: 1139–47.

58. Kugiyama K, Ota Y, Sugiyama S *et al.* Prognostic value of plasma levels of secretory type II phospholipase A2 in patients with unstable angina pectoris. *Am J Cardiol* 2000; **86**: 718–22.

59. Ishihara M, Sato H, Tateishi H *et al.* Implications of prodromal angina pectoris in anterior wall acute myocardial infarction: acute angiographic findings and long-term prognosis. *J Am Coll Cardiol* 1997; **30**: 970–5.

60. Ottani F, Galvani M, Ferrini D, Nicolini FA. Clinical relevance of prodromal angina before acute myocardial infarction. *Int J Cardiol* 1999; **68 (Supplement 1)**: S103–8.

61. Daly LE, Hickey N, Mulcahy R. Course of angina pectoris after an acute coronary event. *Br Med J* 1986; **293**: 653–6.

62. Sheifer SE, Rathmore SS, Gersh BJ *et al.* Time to presentation with acute myocardial infarction in the elderly: associations with race, sex, and socioeconomic characteristics. *Circulation* 2000; **102**: 1651–6.

63. Cameron AA, Davis KB, Rogers WJ. Recurrence of angina after coronary artery bypass surgery: predictors and prognosis (CASS Registry). Coronary Artery Surgery Study. *J Am Coll Cardiol* 1995; **26**: 895–9.

64. Abramov D, Tamariz MG, Sever JY *et al.* The influence of gender on the outcome of coronary artery bypass surgery. *Ann Thorac Surg* 2000; **70**: 800–5.

65. RITA Trial Participants. Coronary angioplasty versus coronary artery bypass surgery: the Randomised Intervention Treatment of Angina (RITA) trial. *Lancet* 1993; **341**: 573–80.

66. Pocock SJ, Henderson RA, Seed P, Treasure T, Hampton JR. Quality of life, employment status, and anginal symptoms after coronary angioplasty or bypass surgery: 3-year follow-up in the Randomised Intervention Treatment of Angina (RITA) trial. *Circulation* 1996; **94**: 135–42.

67. Mehilli J, Kastrati A, Dirschinger J, Bollwein H, Neumann FJ, Schomig A. Differences in prognostic factors and outcomes between women and men undergoing coronary artery stenting. *J Am Med Assoc* 2000; **284**: 1799–805.

Pathophysiology of angina

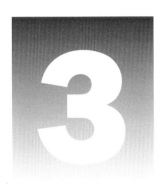

Ross T. Murphy

Introduction

Cardiovascular disease is associated with a significant proportion of premature mortality and morbidity in the developed world. Surveys based on question-naires suggest a UK prevalence of 5–10% in middle-aged men.[1] Ischaemic heart disease (IHD) is the leading cause of premature death in Ireland, with almost double the European Union average for men under 65 years of age. Acute coronary syndromes (ACS), with coronary plaque disruption and/or thrombosis, are the leading causes of hospitalization of adults in the USA, with unstable angina as the principal admission diagnosis, accounting for over 700 000 admissions per year. There is some evidence that the incidence of unstable angina (UA) is increasing, and that it now exceeds that of acute myocardial infarction (AMI).[2]

Surprisingly, almost 50% of these patients will have no classic risk factor (see Box 3.1) for atherosclerosis.[3] The role of several high-profile risk factors (smoking, hypercholesterolaemia, obesity, diabetes and hypertension) in the development of atherosclerosis has received widespread attention, and sig-nificant research over the last decade has advanced the therapeutic responses to such risk factors. However, these factors have only a modest predictive value, and moreover they do not provide a full explanation for the sudden clinical onset of symptoms after the prolonged slow gestation of athero-sclerosis, a disease that manifests after decades of development. There is growing interest in the role of inflammation both in the pathogenesis of atherosclerosis and in acute clinical presentation, particularly of coronary disease. Other well-recognized risk factors (e.g. hyperhomocysteinaemia, hypertriglyceridaemia and poor intake of dietary antioxidants) are starting to have their relative importance defined and their pathophysiological role clari-fied (see Box 3.2). The 'response to injury' hypothesis[4] is the most widely

---

Box 3.1   Classic risk factors for coronary heart disease

1. Hypercholesterolaemia
2. Smoking
3. Diabetes mellitus
4. Hypertension
5. Physical inactivity
6. Obesity

Box 3.2   Emerging risk factors for coronary heart disease

1. Hyperhomocysteinaemia
2. Hypertriglyceridaemia
3. Factor VII activity
4. PAI-1 activity
5. Low circulating levels of antioxidants
6. Fibrinogen
7. Stress/personality type
8. Chronic infections

---

accepted attempt to bring these diverse risk factors together and to present a unified theory of atherosclerosis.

On the basis of intensive research over the last three decades, Ross[4] has attempted to articulate a unifying theory of atherosclerosis as a primarily inflammatory disease. Ross writes that 'the lesions of atherosclerosis represent a series of highly specific cellular and molecular responses that can best be described, in aggregate, as an inflammatory disease'. He also argues against the simplistic notion that low-density-lipoprotein cholesterol (LDL-cholesterol) on its own, by passive accumulation in the vessel wall, causes plaque enlargement and rupture, and he comments on the fact that despite changes in dietary habits and lifestyle, cardiovascular disease continues to be the principal cause of death in the USA, Europe and much of Asia.

Early atheroma

The earliest lesion in atherosclerosis occurs in children and young adults in the form of a fatty streak, and is a purely inflammatory lesion consisting of monocyte-derived macrophages and T-lymphocytes (see Figure 3.1). The formation of such a lesion may result from subtle endothelial dysfunction.

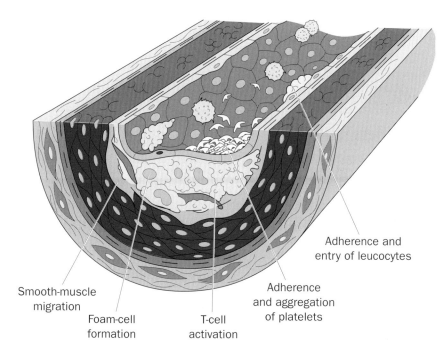

Smooth-muscle
migration

Foam-cell
formation

T-cell
activation

Adherence
and aggregation
of platelets

Adherence and
entry of leucocytes

Figure 3.1
Fatty-streak formation in atherosclerosis. Fatty streaks initially consist of lipid-laden monocytes and macrophages (foam cells) together with T-lymphocytes. Later they are joined by various numbers of smooth muscle cells. The steps involved in this process include the following: smooth muscle migration, which is stimulated by platelet-derived growth factor, fibroblast growth factor 2 and transforming growth factor (beta); T-cell activation, which is mediated by tumour necrosis factor (alpha), interleukin-2 and granulocyte–macrophage colony-stimulating factor; foam-cell formation, which is mediated by oxidized low-density lipoprotein, macrophage colony-stimulating factor, tumour necrosis factor (alpha) and interleukin-1; platelet adherence and aggregation, which are stimulated by integrins, P-selectin, fibrin, thromboxane A_2, and tissue factor, responsible for the adherence and migration of leucocytes. Reproduced with permission. Ross R. Atherosclerosis – an inflammatory disease (review). *N Engl J Med* 1999; **340**: 118.

More severe endothelial dysfunction develops later in life in response to diabetes, cigarette smoking, dyslipidaemia, hypertension, hyperhomocysteinaemia and perhaps infection with *Chlamydia pneumoniae*, cytomegalovirus (CMV), herpes viridiae or a combination of these and other factors with an appropriate genotype. This concept of genetic susceptibility to inflammatory insult is critical to our understanding of early atherosclerosis, and the precise mechanisms are now beginning to be elucidated.

The endothelial responses to these insults are complex and multifaceted, starting with changes in the adhesion of and permeability to platelets and leucocytes, with early infiltration of the endothelial wall by macrophages and specific subtypes of T-lymphocytes.[5] Further inflammation leads to multiplication of the fixed inflammatory population of cells, and migration of more circulating leucocytes to the region. These cells release cytokines, hydrolytic enzymes and growth factors, such as platelet-derived growth factor B and insulin-like growth factor 1, which lead to further inflammation and a perpetuation of the inflammatory cycle. These phases of accumulation and proliferation result in enlargement and remodelling of the plaque, which gives rise to the mature irregular advanced plaque of the adult lesion. An initial compensatory dilatation of the vessel to preserve lumen size[6] is ultimately not enough to prevent a mature flow-limiting stenosis from emerging. The mechanism of such plaque development and its sudden destabilization or fissuring have been the subject of intense scrutiny for over 30 years, and a clearer picture of how risk factors interact with the endothelium to produce athero-sclerosis is now beginning to emerge.

Risk factors and the endothelium

LDL-CHOLESTEROL

Hypercholesterolaemia was identified by the Framingham data as a substantial risk factor for the subsequent development of coronary disease. Brown and Goldstein[7] showed that LDL-cholesterol needs to be modified in order to be rendered atherogenic. LDL-cholesterol may be modified by oxidation, glycation or incorporation into immune complexes. Oxidized LDL can be internalized by macrophages by means of specific scavenger receptors. This internalization leads to the accumulation of lipid peroxides and cholesterol esters, with the resultant formation of foam cells. A recent elegant study illustrated this process in an *in-vivo* experiment in which patients undergoing carotid endarterectomy were injected with radiolabelled autologous native LDL particles 24 h before operation. Their carotid arterial plaques were examined by autoradiography and the LDL was found to be localized predominantly in the foam cells of the atherosclerotic plaque cap and shoulder, with minimal accumulation in the lipid core.[8] Antibodies to oxidized LDL react to the antigens of an atherosclerotic plaque, and patients with clinically proven atherosclerosis have circulating antibodies that react against oxidized LDL. Modified LDL can also induce free-radical formation, a process that can be inhibited by antioxidants such as vitamin E.[9] Modified LDL is also chemotactic for monocytes, and can upregulate the expression of genes for macrophage-colony-stimulating factor (MCSF) and monocyte chemotactic protein (MCP-1).[10] The inflammatory response itself can in turn alter the way in which the endothelium binds to lipoproteins. Tumour necrosis factor-α (TNF-α), interleukin-1 and MCSF increase the binding of LDL to endothelium and also increase transcription of the LDL-receptor gene.[11] After binding to appropriate receptors, LDL can induce expression of interleukin-1.[12] Thus a vicious cycle of inflammation, LDL incorporation and inflammation can be set in motion.

HYPERTENSION

Systemic hypertension is now a well-substantiated risk factor for the development of coronary disease. Data from the Framingham Study and other epidemiological studies show a direct relationship between baseline blood pressure and the incidence of coronary death. Every 7.5 mmHg rise in diastolic pressure is associated with a 29% increase in the risk of coronary disease.[13] Angiotensin II levels are elevated in hypertension, and this molecule, as well as being a potent vasoconstrictor, can cause smooth muscle hypertrophy, increase smooth muscle lipo-oxygenase activity and lead to the increased formation of hydrogen peroxide and other free radicals such as superoxide anion and hydroxyl ions, which are detected in the plasma of patients with hypertension.[14] Patients with an activated renin–angiotensin system (RAS) are at increased risk of acute myocardial infarction, and angiotension II, angiotensin I and angiotensin-converting enzyme (ACE) are expressed at strategic sites in vulnerable coronary plaques. Hypertension may also lead to increased inflammatory activity. Angiotensin II induces interleukin-6 (Il-6) in smooth muscle cells, and is found colocalized to Il-6 in the atherosclerotic coronary arteries of patients undergoing transplantation.[15] Il-6 contributes to the development of atherosclerosis by stimulating the synthesis of matrix-degrading enzymes, LDL receptors and LDL uptake. It is also a central regulator of inflammation and macrophage differentiation. This is consistent with the idea that the activated RAS may stimulate inflammation within the vascular wall and contributes to the development of coronary disease.

DIABETES MELLITUS

Diabetes is a well-established risk factor for cardiovascular disease. It induces endothelial dysfunction and macrovascular disease in a number of ways that are still poorly delineated. Sustained exposure of proteins to hyperglycaemia results in non-enzymatic glycation and the formation of advanced glycosylation end-products (AGE), which may function as signalling pathways to alter vascular function. Reactive oxygen species that are formed during the glycation process may act to inhibit nitric oxide and damage DNA.[16] Glycated lipoproteins are more readily oxidized. Glycated proteins and insulin both stimulate smooth muscle proliferation. Hyperglycaemia increases diacylglycerol levels in vascular tissues. Diacylglycerol is a cofactor for activation of protein kinase C, which is a key regulator of many important vascular functions which are deranged in diabetes, including cell growth, proliferation, adhesion and hyper-coagulability (see Figure 3.2). The increased oxidative stress that is inherent in the diabetic state is associated with over-expression of cell adhesion molecules, and pro-inflammatory cytokines such as TNF-α. Diabetics also have high levels of the procoagulant plasminogen activator inhibitor-1 (PAI-1). Diabetic vasculature may be hyper-responsive to the atherogenic effects of angiotensin II, a potent vasoconstrictor, and stimulation of smooth muscle cell proliferation. Intriguingly, recent trials seem to show that ACE inhibitors not only lower cardiovascular morbidity and mortality,[17] but may also reduce the incidence of diabetes mellitus in a high-risk population. The reasons for such an unexpected

Figure 3.2
Biochemical changes and vascular cell abnormalities associated with hyperglycaemia. Extracellular glucose can glycate proteins without enzyme action and generate oxidative by-products. Glycated proteins accumulate in the extracelluar matrix and bind to advanced glycosylated end-products (AGE) and reporters (AGE-R) expressed on the cell surface. Glycolysis is the major pathway of glucose metabolism in the cell. Increased concentrations of glycolytic metabolites contribute to the *de-novo* synthesis and increased amounts of diacylglycerol – the activating cofactor for protein kinase C (PKC). Signals generated via PKC have been implicated in various diabetic vascular abnormalities. Reproduced with permission from Feener and King. *Lancet* 1997; **350** (Suppl. 1): 9–11.

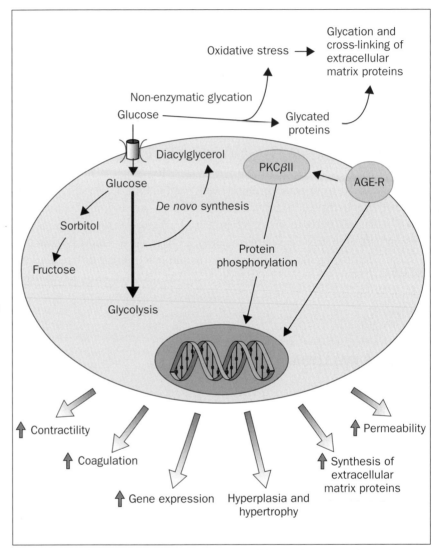

finding are unclear, but may point to the renin-angiotensin system as a central pathway in diabetic risk.

Intensive control of sugars may lessen macrovascular complications in diabetes, but does not abolish the risk, and type II diabetics have the same cardiovascular risk status as those patients with prior myocardial infarction. Obesity, inactivity and the insulin resistance syndrome all contribute to impaired vascular reactivity and endothelial dysfunction. Ongoing work may clarify the role of oxidative stress, cytokine activation and inflammation in diabetic macrovascular disease, but much of the pathophysiology remains poorly understood.

HOMOCYSTEINE

Hyperhomocysteinaemia can be associated with advanced premature athero-sclerosis, and in children who are homozygous for specific genetic defects in homocysteine metabolism (e.g. the enzymes methyltetrahydrofolate reductase and cystathione beta-synthase), aggressive atherosclerotic lesions appear in childhood and the early teens. Levels of homocysteine above the 95th centile carried a relative risk of myocardial infarction of 2.7 in asymptomatic men in the US Physicians Study.[18] Homocysteine, as well as being prothrombotic, is toxic to endothelium, and accelerates smooth muscle cell proliferation. Such endothelial injury results in a pro-inflammatory cascade.[19] Lowering homocysteine levels has been shown to improve endothelial dysfunction, and a number of intervention trials with homocysteine-lowering agents such as folate are ongoing.

INFECTIONS

Controversy about the role that specific infections may play in the development of atherosclerosis has grown during the last decade, and the issue deserves mention here. The hypothesis that infectious agents may cause atherosclerosis was formulated as early as 1911,[20] but received little further attention as a serious concept until the 1970s, when Fabricant *et al.*[21] conducted a series of experiments in which chickens were infected with an avian herpes virus, resulting in the production of florid vascular lesions very similar to the lesions of human atherosclerosis. Subsequent investigators have produced conflicting evidence that a number of infectious agents may be involved in the development of clinically apparent IHD. The infections for which the best evidence has accumulated are *Chlamydia pneumoniae*, *Helicobacter pylori*, certain herpes viridiae and CMV. These agents may have a role as part of a chronic active infection or an acute infection inducing profound immunological activation. They may act as opportunistic agents on a damaged endothelial surface, or merely represent 'innocent bystanders'. Finally, the antigenic isolation of certain agents may merely be a function of antigenic cross-reactivity, a potential flaw in the various tests.

There are two distinct lines of evidence linking infection and atherosclerosis. First, the agent may have been detected in an atherosclerotic plaque via immunocytochemistry or molecular biology techniques. Second, epidemiological data have identified certain agents based on the association between serological positivity and the incidence of disease. Unfortunately, very few data are prospective in nature, and most represent observational data from survivors of incident disease. It has been pointed out that such data represent cross-sectional positive serology at a single point in time, shed little light on the time-scale of the interaction, and may be confounded by the known association with other risk factors, such as smoking.[22] However, CMV infection has been prospectively associated with carotid intima medial thickening over a 20-year period in one study.[23] *Chlamydia pneumoniae* (*Cp*) infection, as represented by anti-*Cp* antibodies in the serum of 220 male survivors of myocardial infarction, was shown to be associated with cardiovascular events over a mean follow-up period of 18 months.[24] *Cp* antigens have been identified in other vascular beds apart from the coronary tree, and are found in carotid and peripheral vascular plaques.[25]

Chronic, asymptomatic infection with *Chlamydia pneumoniae* may be common, with 40–50% of the adult population in Western countries having detectable antibody levels. Intriguing data associate macrolide antibiotic therapy in those post-myocardial infarction patients with high *Cp* titres with a decrease in cardiovascular morbidity,[26] but these findings have been challenged by equivocal results from the ACADEMIC study investigators.[27] *Cp* elementary antibodies and DNA have been demonstrated within atheromatous coronary arteries,[28] and the proposed mechanistic links include macrophage activation (thus triggering an inflammatory process) or a procoagulant state (via increased tissue factor expression). The bacterial lipopolysaccharide cell wall may itself directly damage the endothelial wall. The life cycle of *Cp*, which is an obligate intracellular pathogen, is of particular interest in this context. *Cp* can achieve a state of chronic, intracellular infection in which the bacteria remain viable but do not seem to replicate. This state of 'suspended animation' can be induced by cytokines such as interferon-γ, a product of activated T-lymphocytes within human atheromatous plaques.

Cp is known to produce large amounts of heat shock protein (HSP) during chronic persistent infections. HSP, also known as a chaperonin, is a highly conserved protein whose expression increases during a variety of cell insults, including infection, inflammation, nutritional deprivation and heat shock. HSP acts to stabilize intracellular proteins[29] and can provoke an auto-immune response – a response that has been proposed as a potential promoter of atherosclerosis. Recently, antibodies to HSP have been shown to be associated with an adverse outcome in a prospective study.[30] *Cp* and HSP 60 were found to co-localize in the atheromatous plaques in aortic and carotid specimens that had been surgically removed.[31] This latter study found that *Cp* and HSP both stimulated TNF-α and matrix metalloproteinase activity, thus providing potential mechanisms for the propagation of pro-inflammatory and degradative pathways after *Cp* infection. However, the authors admit that the available data do not yet allow the conclusion that *Cp* infection, which is usually focal and discrete, is a definite primary risk factor for the development of coronary disease.

Local infections with *Cp* may potentiate pre-existing lesions, engender chronic macrophage activation, or be unconnected to the underlying disorder. An intriguing recent report has linked circulating *Cp* antibody immunocomplexes to high lipoprotein(a) levels. Whilst no association was noted between *Cp* antibody status and the incidence of AMI, the authors postulated that *Cp* antibodies could form immunocomplexes with some lipoprotein(a) epitopes that are cross-reactive with *Cp* antigen.[32] These data may represent supportive evidence for an autoimmune process at the centre of the pathogenesis of atherosclerosis. Circulating immunocomplexes also have a tendency to attract and bind complement, initiating an inflammatory cascade. Fibrinogen may be one potential link between infection and the inflammatory response in patients with IHD. The presence of antibodies to *Cp* and to *H. pylori* is associated with high levels of circulating fibrinogen, and one recent study showed a reduction of fibrinogen levels in patients treated with short courses of conventional antibiotics for these two common infections against a background of chronic IHD.[33]

However, the data linking *H. pylori* to coronary events are less conclusive. Quinn *et al.*[34] studied the relationship between angiographically documented coronary disease and serological evidence of *H. pylori* infection, and after adjusting for confounding variables, in particular socio-economic class, found no association among 488 patients attending for coronary angiogram (odds ratio 1.3, 95% confidence interval 0.83–2.16). A weak association was diluted by a similar adjustment in another study of the relationship between high-virulence *H. pylori* and myocardial infarction in 259 myocardial infarction survivors and matched controls.[35] The seminal retrospective study that initially reported the link (a fourfold increase in the risk of coronary disease in seropositive men) was limited by its size and retrospective nature,[36] and has been contradicted by subsequent larger studies. The proposed link was built on the observation that *H. pylori* positivity conferred a risk of elevated fibrinogen levels, and elevated indices of inflammation, e.g. C-reactive protein (CRP), but this has not been borne out by more recent studies.

In summary, chronic infection has a possible role in the pathogenesis of atherosclerosis, but the accumulated evidence does not allow the establishment of a definite causal link. More data, both on the serological connection and on the mechanisms of interaction, are needed before a definitive connection can be made.

Shear stress

Vascular shear stress is another proposed initiator of the atheromatous plaque. In this case the emphasis is not on the humoral/biochemical stimuli to endothelial activation, but rather on the consequences of haemodynamic stress and hydrostatic pressures in a pulsatile blood vessel.[37] Striking changes in cell shape, cell alignment and cytoskeletal architecture occur in laminar flow models using endothelial cell lines, including subtle changes in membrane deformability and cell division rate.[38] These may be viewed as *in-vitro* adaptations, and the process involves alterations in the expression of such cell-surface adhesion molecules as platelet endothelial cell adhesion molecule-1 (PECAM-1). Some of these effects are analogous to the stimulation of endothelial cells by cytokines. For instance, when cultured human umbilical vein endothelial cells (HUVEC) are exposed to steady lateral shear stress, there is a time-dependent induction of intercellular adhesion molecule-1 (ICAM-1), which is evident at mRNA level by 2 h and detectable as a functional membrane protein as long as 48 h after exposure to the shear stress.[39]

This enhanced expression in part reflected increased transcription, and did not result in increased expression of either vascular cell adhesion molecule-1 (VCAM-1) or endothelial selectin (E-selectin) in this model. Indeed, in one murine cell model, shear stress preconditioning down-regulated VCAM-1 expression, illustrating the complexity of biomechanical interaction.[40] Monocyte chemotactic protein-1 (MCP-1), an important chemokine *in vivo*, was seen to be up-regulated under shear flow stress conditions.[41] *In-vivo* experiments in rabbit carotid arteries revealed a similar pattern of ICAM-1 and VCAM-1 up-regulation in response to surgically induced alterations in flow dynamics.[42] Gimbrone *et al.*[37] have argued that the best evidence for flow-induced inflammatory change in the vascular endothelium comes from the non-random distribution of early lesions of atherosclerosis in primates and humans, at bifurcations, abrupt curves and sharp bends. Thus *in vivo* the endothelial surface is subject to significant biomechanical stresses, the response to which, in many cases, mimics the response to pro-inflammatory cytokine stimulation, and is accompanied by significant up-regulation of endothelial adhesion molecules and leucocyte/endothelial interactions.

Endothelial injury and ongoing inflammation: the mechanism for plaque development?

The diverse risk factors associated with coronary artery disease may share a final common pathway in the induction of endothelial gene expression.[43] Oxidative stress and a number of other endothelial insults may act via secondary messengers to activate the key pro-inflammatory stimulator nuclear factor kappa B (NFκB). The proteins of the NFκB family form inactive heterodimeric compounds in the cytoplasm with IκB, inhibitors of nuclear translocation, in many cell types, including T-lymphocytes, monocytes, macrophages, endothelial cells and smooth muscle cells, which dissociate on stimulation and then activate a variety of pro-inflammatory genes. Activators of NFκB include lipopolysaccharide (LPS), interleukin-1 (IL-1) and tumour necrosis factor-α (TNF-α). NFκB is also sensitive to oxidative stress *in vitro* and *in vivo*. Once translocated, NFκB activates genes involved in the immune and inflammatory response and allows the production of IL-1, IL-6, IL-8, interferon and TNF-α, as well as cell adhesion molecules (CAMs) such as VCAM-1, ICAM-1 and E-selectin. NFκB also regulates expression of the genes that encode it and IκB, and is thus capable of self-regulation.[44] The major NFκB family members have been isolated, including the precursors p105 and p100, and the factors Re1A(p65), Re1B, c-Rel, NFκB1(p50) and NFκB2(p52). In many instances, NFκB functions as a heterodimer of 50-kDa protein.

Specific members of the NFκB family may be selectively activated. Using electromobility gel shift assays (EMSA), it has been shown that the NFκB members p50, p52, p65, c-Rel and RelB were expressed in balloon-injured rabbit carotid arteries,[45] that such activation coincides with smooth muscle proliferative phases and that it is accompanied by a dramatic reduction in the inhibitor proteins Iκα, Iκβ and p105. Subsequent to this activation, VCAM-1 and monocyte chemotactic protein-1 (MCP-1) were induced in smooth muscle and endothelial cells, with increased monocyte adhesion as early as 4 h after injury in this model. This monocyte adhesion may provide an important clue as to why there are lipid-laden macrophages at the core of the atherosclerotic plaque and how they got there. Another model suggested that functionally active NFκB is found in the nuclear extracts of cultured endothelial cells on exposure to activated platelets,[46] which also showed significant expression of MCP-1 and ICAM-1 after such exposure. Furthermore, transfection of cells with appropriate inhibitory NFκB oligonucleotides resulted in nuclear localization of these nucleotides and a subsequent decrease in MCP-1 and ICAM-1 production upon exposure to activated platelets.

MCP-1 is a small, inducible secreted pro-inflammatory chemotactic cytokine. It has *in-vitro* and *in-vivo* ability to chemoattract monocytes, and it also has the reported ability to stimulate degranulation and respiratory burst in monocytes. MCP-1 has been implicated as an important mediator of monocyte and T-cell infiltration in a variety of inflammatory conditions. The role of MCP-1 in atherosclerosis has come under extensive scrutiny recently. During the development of atherosclerosis, MCP-1 functions by recruiting monocytes into the subendothelial layer, and it is considered to be critical for the initiation and enlargement of plaques.[47] MCP-1 is a potent chemoattractant for monocytes, and ICAM-1 in this context mediates leucocyte adhesion to the endothelium via fibrinogen and the integrins Mac-1 (CD11b/18) and LFA-4 (CD49d). Serum MCP-1 levels have been reported to be elevated in patients with AMI.[48] Oxidized LDL-cholesterol is considered

Figure 3.3

Pathways by which vascular and extravascular sources of inflammation result in circulating levels of serum markers that provide a reflection of the underlying inflammatory response. Inflammation (systemic or local, either in the blood vessel itself or elsewhere) triggers the production of multipotent pro-inflammatory cytokines that we denote here as 'primary' (e.g. IL-1β or TNF-α). These primary cytokines can directly elicit production by endothelial and other cells of adhesion molecules, procoagulants and other mediators that may be released in soluble form into circulating blood. Primary cytokines also stimulate the production of 'messenger' cytokine, IL-6, which induces expression of hepatic genes encoding acute-phase reactants found in blood, including C-reactive protein (CRP) and serum amyloid-A (SAA). Thus these markers in serum can provide a window on the inflammatory status of the individual, that is otherwise inaccessible in the intact subject. Reproduced with permission of the American Heart Association from Libby et al. Circulation 1999; **100**: 1149.

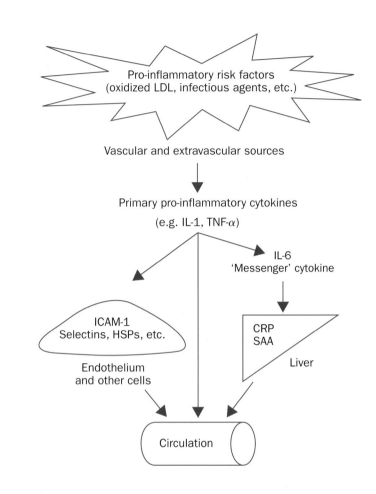

to be antigenic and is incorporated into macrophages and monocytes in the arterial intima. When LDL-deficient mice were fed a high-cholesterol diet it was noted that those mice which were also MCP-1 deficient deposited less LDL and had fewer macrophages in their aortic walls.[49]

The response of the cell to NFκB release is twofold, as outlined above, involving both CAM activation and secretory molecule release (see Figure 3.3). The inflammatory response is associated with the generation of cytokines that act on the local endothelial cell wall and the induction and expression of CAMs. CAMs may have a direct role in the pathogenesis of atherosclerosis.[50] Davies et al.[51] observed CAM staining on the endothelial surface of atherosclerotic coronary arteries. VCAM-1 staining was found only on diseased artery, and E-selectin was found on both fibrous and lipid-containing plaques.[51] These CAMs play a central role in the attraction and adhesion of monocytes and neutrophils to the endothelial wall and their subsequent 'rolling' or transendothelial migration across the arterial intima.[52]

CAMs are an essential component of the inflammatory response. Transgenic mice with CAM knockout genes die early in life from overwhelming sepsis, as they are unable to localize leucocytes to the interstitium. The four principal molecules of note have only been individually characterized in the last decade, and they include ICAM-1, VCAM-1, E-selectin and platelet selectin (P-selectin). Analysis of the endothelial CAM genes has revealed putative NFκB binding sites in the 5′ flanking sequences.[43] A complex sequence of stimulation and autoregulation stimulates transcription of the VCAM-1, ICAM-1 and E-selectin genes, with a consequent functional increase in endothelial/leucocyte binding seen in early atherosclerosis. Activation of the genes for soluble cytokines, such as MCP-1 and GM-CSF, results in monocyte recruitment and localization.

Thus a variety of specific stimuli for NFκB activation exist, including oxidative stress, inflammatory cytokines, oxidized LDL, smoking, and the advanced glycosylation end-products (AGE) of diabetes mellitus. This pathway also provides a mechanistic explanation for the putative association between certain infective agents, such as CMV and herpes viridiae, which are known activators of NFκB,[53] and atherosclerosis. In summary, Collins and White[43] propose NFκB as 'necessary, but not sufficient' for inflammatory up-regulation in the dysfunctional endothelium, which might act as a final common pathway for the multiplicity of risk factors in developing the atherosclerotic plaque.

Acute coronary syndromes

Significant research that has accumulated over the last decade suggests that inflammation may be of fundamental importance in the acute clinical expression of coronary heart disease. A growing body of evidence supports the hypothesis that atherosclerosis shows many similarities to other autoimmune/ inflammatory diseases, and there are surprising similarities between the immunological response of the body to the prototype of autoimmune disease, namely rheumatoid arthritis, and the response to chronic atherosclerosis. These responses are even more striking in unstable coronary disease. The initial evidence for this came from histological studies, both from postmortem series and from atherectomy specimens collected *in vivo*. Van der Wal *et al.*[54] described the site of intimal rupture or erosion as being characterized by an inflammatory process regardless of the dominant plaque morphology or superimposed thrombus. They found that the number of lesions on atherectomy specimens which contained recently activated T-lymphocytes (and were interleukin-2-receptor positive) increased with the clinical severity of the coronary syndrome, so that 52% of stable angina patients were staining positive, compared with 77.8% of stabilized unstable angina plaques,

Figure 3.4
Plaque stability: a dynamic model. Reproduced with permission of the American Heart Association. From Libby. *Circulation* 1995; **91**: 2844–50.

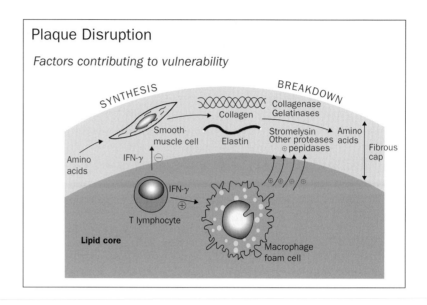

90.9% of refractory unstable angina plaques and 89.5% of AMI plaques. Likewise, macrophage infiltration has been consistently observed in plaques from patients presenting with acute coronary syndromes.[55] These macrophages drive an inflammatory process that involves production of the degradatory matrix metalloproteinases (MMPs) and the induction of smooth muscle cell apoptosis.[38] Libby[56] established the concept of plaque cap as a dynamic entity, with collagen synthesis balanced by collagen degradation (see Figure 3.4). Loss of smooth muscle cells reduces collagen production, but in the acute setting, lymphocyte-derived interferon-γ may be more important in actively suppressing collagen synthesis and thus weakening the plaque cap. Apo-E-deficient mice that lack the interferon-γ receptor have markedly diminished atherosclerotic lesions.[24] Similarly, activation of macrophages by TNF-α leads to MMP production and enhanced lytic activity in the vulnerable plaque cap. Both of these axes are activated in the acute coronary syndromes.

The occurrence of plaque disruption by rupture or fissuring in a coronary artery does not appear to be related to the severity of lumen stenosis. It is now known from incidental angiographic series that 70% of all acute occlusions occur from a stenosis that is less than 50% of the vessel diameter. Fissuring of coronary plaques is absent in 25–40% of patients who are dying with a clinical diagnosis of acute coronary syndromes, and up to 25% of patients in one postmortem series who were dying of non-cardiac causes had coronary plaque fissuring as an incidental finding. Thus *de-novo* mechanical plaque disruption may not account for all of the features of clinical presentation of acute coronary disease. Inflammatory change is an almost universal histological finding in atherectomy and post-mortem specimens, and the pathophysiological reasons for the sudden destabilization of these plaques are poorly understood.

The process that leads to plaque instability and rupture may depend on a number of factors, including plaque composition, cap strength, core composition, local vasoconstriction and thrombosis.

Libby[56] has highlighted three fundamentals factors for plaque stability:

1. the fibrous content of the plaque cap;
2. the lipid content and size of the core;
3. the relative paucity of smooth muscle cells in the vicinity.

Accelerated degradation of the fibrous plaque and in particular of collagen may contribute to plaque weakening. The large molecules that constitute the extracellular matrix in an arterial wall usually exhibit considerable metabolic stability. Collagen turnover is normally quite slow, and forms a triple helical structure that is a robust defence against many proteolytic enzymes. The activity of the degrading MMP enzymes plays an important role in plaque instablility. MMPs are part of a proteolytic superfamily of digestive enzymes that includes interstitial collagenase, gelatinases and stromelysins. These enzyme systems work extracellularly and at physiological pH. Collagenases can cleave the normally protease-resistant fibrillar collagens that do so much to strengthen the fibrous cap, the gelatinases break down collagen fragments, and the stromelysins degrade the larger proteoglycan molecules, and may also break down elastin, an important structural element of the extracellular matrix. The major regulators of MMP activity in normal physiological circumstances are the tissue inhibitors of metalloproteinases (TIMPs), which have been the focus of intensive study during the last decade. Normal vascular tissue seems to express variable amounts of TIMPs constitutively, but pro-inflammatory cytokines such as TNF-α and interleukin-1 (IL-1) up-regulate degradatory enzymes such as collagenase, gelatinase B and stromelysin, which are not normally expressed under basal conditions. Importantly, *in-vitro* experiments using these cytokines do not appear to up-regulate the inhibitory TIMP system. Thus pro-inflammatory stimuli can lead to human atherosclerotic plaques with an excess of matrix-degrading activity and unopposed enzymatic activity in the vulnerable plaque. In these diseased areas, macrophages, T-cells and smooth muscle cells all express more interstitial collagenase, stromelysin and gelatinase activity than normal artery, especially in the shoulder region of vulnerable plaques (see Plate 3.1).

Another factor in the clinical presentation of coronary disease is the impaired responsiveness of diseased parts of coronary vessels to basally released endothelial-dependent vasodilators. Much research during the last decade has focused on this failure to respond to vasospasm. The key mediator of this response is nitric oxide (NO) or endothelium-derived relaxing factor (EDRF), and impaired production of and response to this potent locally produced vasodilator play a significant role in the presentation of angina. Damaged endothelial tissue shows both decreased secretion and decreased responsiveness to NO, which normally activates guanylate cyclase to increase intracellular cGMP levels, with a fall in intracellular calcium levels and a consequent relaxation of smooth muscle tone. NO has also been shown to inhibit platelet aggregation and suppress the proliferation of vascular smooth muscle cells.

Inflammatory markers

If inflammation is important in the pathophysiology of atherosclerosis, the pattern of inflammatory marker expression may be a useful way of monitoring disease progress. Braunwald characterized the markers of inflammation as still 'primitive' but 'of growing interest and utility'.[57] C-reactive protein (CRP), an acute-phase protein that is produced by the liver in response to interleukin-6 (IL-6), is a well-established marker of acute and chronic inflammatory states.[58] Long utilized as a non-specific marker of generalized inflammation, vasculitis or neoplasia, it has recently attracted attention as a specific disease-activity marker, playing a part in as yet poorly defined pathological paradigms. Particular attention has been focused on the role of modest elevations in CRP levels in predicting future cardiovascular events, and it has been proposed as a new prognostic marker in atherosclerosis.

New, high-sensitivity CRP assays have emerged during the last decade, and a number of independent studies have now found statistical associations between atherosclerosis and levels of CRP which would until now have been regarded as high-normal range. Data from the US Physicians Health Study[59] show that apparently healthy men with CRP levels in the highest quartile had a threefold risk of developing future myocardial infarction (relative risk 2.9, $P < 0.001$) and twice the risk of developing stroke (relative risk 1.9, $P < 0.02$) compared with men with levels in the lowest quartile. These risks were calculated over a 10-year follow-up, and were independent of traditional risk factors such as smoking, lipid and fibrinogen levels. A nested case–control study from a Danish population found that modest increases in CRP were present for up to 15 years prior to the onset of clinically overt coronary disease.[60] The Helsinki Heart Study, a primary prevention trial that is now nearly a decade old, recently showed a combined relative risk of coronary death or myocardial infarction of 25.4 for subjects with elevated levels of both CRP and antibody titres to *Chlamydia pneumoniae* and herpes simplex 1, bringing together the infectious and inflammatory hypotheses in an intriguing combination.[61]

CRP levels are elevated in patients with stable angina compared with controls,[62] and a linear relationship between CRP levels and progressive complexity of disease was noted in a large cohort of patients post myocardial infarction.[63] Similarly, CRP is associated with an increased risk of future ischaemic events in survivors of myocardial infarction, and this predictive value is additive to that of total cholesterol levels.[64] Increased CRP levels were associated with a poorer outcome at 1 year in patients who had survived a first uncomplicated myocardial infarction. These were patients without residual ischaemia on exercise testing, and with normal left ventricular function, and in a Cox regression model for a number of variables, only elevated CRP levels were independently related to subsequent cardiac events.[65]

The role of CRP as a marker of potential instability in acute coronary syndromes has only recently been established. A substudy of the FRISC trial found that high CRP levels were associated with an adverse outcome in patients presenting with unstable angina.[66] This observation has been reaffirmed in several other studies. Long-term follow-up (mean period 37 months) in the FRISC group showed initial CRP levels to be a strong independent predictor of mortality. Death rates in patients with CRP levels of <2 mg/L, 2–10 mg/L and >10 mg/L were 5.7%, 7.8% and 16.5%, respectively.[67] CRP levels at the time of discharge in patients with unstable angina have been shown to be elevated in some cases after the waning of symptoms, and these elevations were associated with a higher medium-term event rate,[68] also supporting the hypothesis that these markers represent ongoing background inflammation. CRP level at the time of discharge was the strongest independent predictor of increased 90-day risk of recurrent angina, myocardial infarction or death (see Figure 3.5).[69]

Elevated CRP levels are a marker of increased production of IL-1 and IL-6. CRP itself can activate monocytes to produce tissue factor, activate complement and induce monocyte and endothelial release of IL-1 and IL-6. The latter two cytokines have intrinsic prothrombotic properties, but the mechanisms that lead to elevated CRP levels may be multifactorial, and despite extensive research they remain poorly understood. Some authorities propose a central role for IL-6, in that it is a powerful regulator of the hepatic acute-phase response. IL-6 also decreases lipoprotein lipase activity and increases macrophage uptake of lipids. It has been expressed in macrophage foam cells and vascular smooth muscle cells in the cap and shoulder regions of vulnerable plaques, and in fatty streaks.[70] The hepatic acute-phase response includes paracrine and autocrine activation of monocytes, elevated levels of plasma fibrinogen, plasma viscosity, increased platelet number and activity, and direct stimulation of CRP. Although CRP has attracted much attention as a stable reliable marker with a WHO-accepted standard assay, it is possible that it merely represents the stable surrogate marker of IL-6 and other cytokine activity. IL-1 has a very short half-life in serum, and Il-6 assays have only been widely available in the last decade. IL-6 has been

Figure 3.5
Kaplan–Meier plot: cumulative freedom from risk of death, myocardial infarction or refractory angina within 90 days in patients with CRP levels above or below 1.5 mg/dL. Reproduced with permission of the American Heart Association. From Ferreiros *et al. Circulation* 1999; **100**: 1958–63.

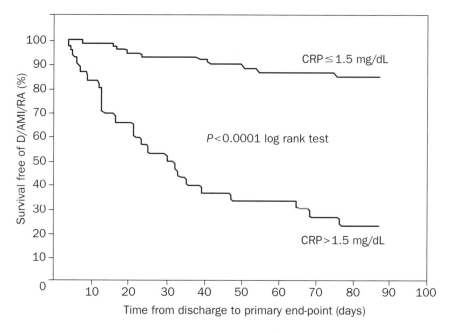

shown to be elevated in a number of studies in patients with unstable angina,[71] to have similar prognostic significance to CRP, and to have a measurable transcardiac gradient in one invasive study of patients undergoing coronary angioplasty for ongoing clinical instability.[72]

CAMs may also act as peripheral markers of central disease. The extracellular portion of these molecules is enzymatically cleaved in a stereotyped manner, or alternatively it is spliced and then shed into the peripheral circulation, where it can be measured in serum or plasma as a soluble cell adhesion molecule (sCAM). sCAMs from the peripheral circulation can be used experimentally to follow the course of disease in a number of inflammatory disorders. They may also be useful for following the pattern of endothelial dysfunction and possibly the glycaemic control of patients with insulin-dependent diabetes mellitus.[73] sCAMs are predictive of ischaemic events in healthy men (US Physicians Health Study).[64] The levels of soluble CAMs have been shown to be elevated in acute coronary syndromes, and to predict events in patients with stable angina.[74] Recent work has shown that the levels of soluble VCAM-1 were predictive of 6-month recurrent ischaemic events in patients with unstable angina.[75] Thus a number of interlinked inflammatory markers may help to predict outcome in patients with acute coronary syndromes. The main impact of these observations has been to help explore further the pathogenesis of stable and unstable angina, but it is possible that rapid testing of a combination of markers may be clinically useful in the very near future.

Summary

Coronary artery disease is a complex, multifactorial disorder. It has a long genesis as a silent disease, and it manifests in a number of different ways. Multiple risk factors have been described, and significant new research in the last decade has gone some way towards explaining how these risk factors interact and cause the endothelial dysfunction and plaque build-up which characterize the adult lesions of atherosclerosis. Inflammation seems to play a significant role both in the development of plaque and in the destablization that can precipitate the clinical onset of angina. Our knowledge of the causes of atherosclerosis is still very limited, but the next decade promises exciting developments in both our understanding and our ability to treat the consequences of coronary atheroma.

References

1. Shaper AG, Cook DG, Walker M *et al.* Prevalence of ischaemic heart disease in middle-aged British men. *Br Heart J* 1984; **51**: 595–605.
2. Theroux P, Liddon RM. Unstable angina: pathogenesis, diagnosis and treatment. *Curr Prob Cardiol* 1993; **18**: 157–231.
3. Braunwald E. Shattuck Lecture. Cardiovascular medicine at the turn of the millennium: triumphs, concerns and opportunities. *N Engl J Med* 1997; **337**: 1360–9.
4. Ross R. Atherosclerosis – an inflammatory disease (review). *N Engl J Med* 1999; **340**: 115–221.
5. Jonasson L, Holm J, Skalli O *et al.* Regional accumulation of T-cells, macrophages and smooth muscle cells in the human atherosclerotic plaque. *Arteriosclerosis* 1986; **6**: 131–8.
6. Glagov S. Hemodynamic risk factors, mechanical stress, mural architecture, medial nutrition and the vulnerability of arteries to atherosclerosis. In: *The pathogenesis of atherosclerosis.* Baltimore, MD: Williams and Wilkins, 1972: 164–88.
7. Brown MS, Goldstein JL. Lipoprotein metabolism in the macrophage: implications for cholesterol deposition in atherosclerosis. *Annu Rev Biochem* 1983; **52**: 233–61.
8. Iuliano L, Mauriello A, Sbarigia E *et al.* Radiolabelled native LDL injected into patients with carotid stenosis accumulates in macrophages of atherosclerotic plaques. *Circulation* 2000; **101**: 1249–54.
9. Nunes GL, Robinson K, Kalynch A *et al.* Vitamins C and E inhibit O_2 production in the pig coronary artery. *Circulation* 1997; **96**: 3593–601.
10. Leonard EJ, Toshimura T. Human monocyte chemoattractant protein-1. *Immunol Today* 1990; **11**: 97–101.

11. Stopeck AT, Nicholson AC, Mancini FP *et al.* Cytokine regulation of low-density-lipoprotein receptor gene transcription in Hepg2 cells. *J Biol Chem* 1993; **268**: 17489–94.

12. Palkama T. Induction of interleukin-1 production by ligands binding to the scavenger receptor in human monocytes and the THP-1 cell line. *Immunology* 1991; **74**: 432–8.

13. Braunwald E. Fiftieth Anniversary Article: myocardial oxygen consumption – the quest for its determinants and some clinical fallout. *J Am Coll Cardiol* 2000; **35** (**Supplement E**): B45–8.

14. Griendling KK, Alexander RW. Oxidative stress and cardiovascular disease. *Circulation* 1997; **96**: 3264–5.

15. Scheiffer B, Scheiffer E, Hilfiker-Kleiner D *et al.* Expression of ATII and IL6 in human coronary atherosclerotic plaques. *Circulation* 2000; **101**: 1372–8.

16. Feener EP, King GL. Vascular function in diabetes mellitus. *Lancet* 1997; **350 (Supplement 1)**: SI9–13.

17. The HOPE Study investigators. Effect of angiotensin-converting enzyme inhibitor, ramipril, on cardiovascular outcomes in high-risk patients. *N Engl J Med* 2000; **342**: 145–53.

18. Stampfer MJ, Malinow MR, Willet MC *et al.* A prospective study of plasma homocysteine and risk of myocardial infarction in US physicians. *J Am Med Assoc* 1992; **268**: 877–9.

19. Harker LA, Ross R, Slichter SJ. Homocysteine-induced arteriosclerosis: the role of endothelial cell injury and platelet response in its genesis. *J Clin Invest* 1976; **58**: 731–41.

20. Frothingham C. The relation between acute infectious disease and arterial lesions. *Arch Intern Med* 1911; **8**: 153–62.

21. Fabricant CG, Fabricant J, Litrenta MM *et al.* Virus-induced atherosclerosis. *J Exp Med* 1978; **148**: 335–40.

22. Buja LM. Does atherosclerosis have an infectious aetiology? *Circulation* 1996; **94**: 872–3.

23. Nieto FJ, Adam E, Sorlie P *et al.* Cohort study of CMV infection as a risk factor for carotid intima media thickening: a measure of subclinical atherosclerosis. *Circulation* 1996; **94**: 922–7.

24. Gupta S, Leatham EW, Carrington D *et al.* Elevated *Chlamydia pneumoniae* antibodies, cardiovascular events and azithromycin in male survivors of myocardial infarction. *Circulation* 1997; **96**: 404–7.

25. Ong G, Tomas BJ, Mansfield AO *et al.* Detection and widespread distribution of *Chlamydia pneumoniae* in the vascular system and its possible implications. *J Clin Pathol* 1996; **49**: 102–6.

26. Gurfinkel E, Bozovich G, Daroca A *et al.* Randomised trial of roxithromycin in non-Q-wave coronary syndromes: Roxis pilot study. *Lancet* 1997; **350**: 404–7.

27. Anderson JL, Muhlestein JB, Carlquist J *et al.* Randomized secondary prevention trial of azithromycin in patients with coronary artery disease and serological evidence for *C. pneumoniae* infection: the ACADEMIC study. *Circulation* 1999; **99**: 1540–7.

28. Kuo CC, Shor A, Cambell LA *et al.* Demonstration of *C. pneumoniae* in atherosclerotic lesions of coronary arteries. *J Infect Dis* 1993; **167**: 841–9.

29. Young RA, Eliot TJ. Stress proteins, infection and immune surveillance. *Cell* 1989; **59**: 5–8.

30. Xu Q, Kiehel S, Mayr M *et al.* Association of serum antibodies to hsp 65 with carotid atherosclerosis: clinical significance determined in a follow-up study. *Circulation* 1999; **100**: 1169–74.

31. Kol A, Sukhova GK, Lichtman AH *et al.* Chlamydial heat shock protein 60 localizes in human atheroma and regulates macrophage tumor necrosis factor-alpha and matrix metalloproteinase expression. *Circulation* 1998; **98**: 300–7.

32. Glader CA, Bowman J, Saikuku P *et al.* The proatherogenic properties of lipoprotein(a) may be enhanced through the formation of circulating immunocomplexes containing Cp-specific IgG antibodies. *Eur Heart J* 2000; **21**: 639–46.

33. Torgano G, Cosenti R, Mandelli C *et al.* Treatment of *H. pylori* and *C. pneumoniae* infections decreases fibrinogen plasma levels in patients with ischaemic heart disease. *Circulation* 1999; **99**: 1555–9.

34. Quinn MJ, Foley JB, Mulvihill NT *et al. Helicobacter pylori* serology in patients with angiographically documented coronary artery disease. *Am J Cardiol* 1999; **83**: 1664–6.

35. Murray LJ, Bamford KB, Kee F *et al.* Infection with virulent strains of *H. pylori* is not associated with ischaemic heart disease: evidence from a population-based case–control study of myocardial infarction. *Atherosclerosis* 2000; **149**: 379–85.

36. Whincup P, Danesh J, Walker M *et al.* Prospective study of potentially virulent strains of *H. pylori* and coronary heart disease in middle-aged men. *Circulation* 2000; **101**: 1647–52.

37. Gimbrone MA Jr, Nagel T, Topper JN. Biomechanical activation: an emerging paradigm in endothelial adhesion biology. *J Clin Invest* 1997; **99**: 1809–13.

38. Davies PF. Flow-mediated endothelial mechanotransduction. *Physiol Rev* 1995; **75**: 519–60.

39. Nagel T, Resnick WJ, Atkinsin CF *et al.* Shear stress selectively upregulates ICAM-1 expression in HUVEC cells. *J Clin Invest* 1994; **94**: 885–91.

40. Varner SE, Nerem RM, Medford RM *et al.* Laminar shear stress regulates VCAM-1 expression. *Ann Biochem* 1994; **22**: 40.

41. Lin MC, Almus-Jacobs F, Chen HH *et al.* Shear stress induction of the tissue factor gene. *J Clin Invest* 1997; **99**: 737–44.

42. Walpola PL, Gotlieb AI, Cybulsky MI *et al.* Expression of VCAM-1 and ICAM-1 and monocyte adherence in arteries exposed to altered shear stress. *Arterioscler Thromb Vasc Biol* 1995; **14**: 133–40.

43. Collins KA, White WL. ICAM-1 and bcl-2 are differentially expressed in early evolving malignant melanoma. *Am J Dermopathol* 1995; **17**: 429–38.

44. Ritchie M. NFκB is selectively and markedly activated in humans with unstable angina pectoris. *Circulation* 1998; **98**: 1707–13.

45. Lindner V. The NFκB and IκB system in injured arteries. *Pathobiology* 1998; **66**: 311–20.

46. Gawaz M, Neumann FJ, Dickfield T *et al.* Activated platelets induce MCP-1 secretion and surface expression of intercellular adhesion molecule-1. *Circulation* 1998; **98**: 1164–71.

47. Schwartz CJ. Role of MCP-1 in atherosclerosis. *Clin Cardiol* 1991; **1**: 11.

48. Matsumori A, Furukawa Y, Hashimoto T *et al.* Plasma levels of the monocyte chemotactic and activating factor/monocyte chemoattractant protein-1 are elevated in patients with acute myocardial infarction. *J Mol Cell Cardiol* 1997; **29**: 419–23.

49. Gu L. MCP-1-dependent deposition of LDL in LDL-deficient mice. *Mol Cell Biol* 1998; **2**: 275.

50. Springer TA, Cybulsky MI. Traffic signals on endothelium for leukocytes in health, inflammation and atherosclerosis. In: Fuster V, Ross R, Topol EJ (eds) *Atherosclerosis and coronary artery disease.* Philadelphia, PA: Lippincott-Raven Publishers, 1996: 511–37.

51. Davies MJ, Gordon JL, Gearing AJ *et al.* The expression of the adhesion molecules ICAM-1, VCAM-1, PECAM and E-Selectin in human atherosclerosis. *J Pathol* 1993; **171**: 223–9.

52. Cotran RS, Mayados Norton T. Endothelial molecules in health and disease. *Pathol Biol* 1998; **46**: 164–70.

53. Sambucetti LC, Cherrington JM, Wilkinson GW *et al.* NFκB activation of the CMV enhancer is mediated by a viral transactivator and by T-cell stimulation. *EMBO J* 1989; **8**: 4251–8.

54. Van der Wal AC, Pieck JJ, de Boer OJ. Recent activation of the plaque immune response in coronary lesions underlying acute coronary syndromes. *Heart* 1998; **80**: 14–18.

55. Moreno PR, Falk E, Palacios IF *et al.* Macrophage infiltration in acute coronary syndromes: implications for plaque rupture. *Circulation* 1994; **90**: 775–8.

56. Libby P. The molecular basis of the acute coronary syndromes. *Circulation* 1995; **91**: 2844–50.

57. Braunwald E. Unstable angina: an etiological approach to management. *Circulation* 1998; **98**: 2219–22.

58. Pepys MB. The acute-phase response and C-reactive protein. In: Weatherall DJ, Ledingham JCG, Warrell DA (eds) *Oxford textbook of medicine*. Oxford: Oxford University Press, 1995: 1527–33.

59. Ridker PM, Cushman M, Stampfer MJ *et al.* Inflammation, aspirin, and the risk of cardiovascular disease in apparently healthy men. *N Engl J Med* 1997; **336**: 973–9.

60. Gram J, Bladjberg EM, Moller I *et al.* TPA and CRP in acute coronary disease. A nested case–control study. *J Intern Med* 2000; **247**: 205–12.

61. Roivainen M, Viik-Kajander M, Palosuo T *et al.* Infections, inflammation and the risk of coronary disease. *Circulation* 2000; **101**: 252–7.

62. Haverkate F, Thompson SG, Pyke SDM *et al.* Production of C-reactive protein and risk of coronary events in stable and unstable angina. *Lancet* 1997; **349**: 462–9.

63. Tataru MC, Heinrich J, Junker R *et al.* CRP and the severity of atherosclerosis in myocardial infarction patients with stable angina pectoris. *Eur Heart J* 2000; **21**: 1000–8.

64. Ridker PM, Hennekens CH, Roitman-Johnson B *et al.* Plasma concentrations of sICAM-1 and risks of future myocardial infarction in apparently healthy men. *Lancet* 1998; **351**: 88–92.

65. Tomassi S, Carluccio E, Bentivoglio M *et al.* CRP as a marker for cardiac ischemic events after a first uncomplicated myocardial infarction. *Am J Cardiol* 1999; **83**: 1595–9.

66. Toss L. Prognostic influence of fibrinogen and C-reactive protein levels in unstable coronary heart disease. *Circulation* 1997; **95**: 4204–10.

67. Lindahl B, Toss H, Siegbahn A *et al.* Markers of myocardial damage and inflammation in relation to long-term mortality in unstable coronary artery disease. *N Engl J Med* 2000; **343**: 1139–47.

68. Biasucci LM, Liuzzo G, Grillo RL *et al.* Elevated levels of C-reactive protein at discharge in patients with unstable angina predict recurrent instablility. *Circulation* 1999; **99**: 855–60.

69. Ferreiros ER, Boissonnet CP, Pizarro R *et al.* Independent prognostic value of elevated C-reactive protein in unstable angina. *Circulation* 1999; **100**: 1958–63.

70. Yudkin JS, Kumari M, Humphries SE *et al.* Inflammation, obesity, stress and coronary heart disease: is Il-6 the link? *Atherosclerosis* 1999; **148**: 209–14.

71. Biasucci LM, Vitelli A, Liuzzo G *et al.* Elevated levels of IL-6 in unstable angina. *Circulation* 1996; **94**: 874–7.

72. Cusack M, Marber MS, Odemuyiwa S *et al.* Does myocardial necrosis contribute to the inflammatory response in unstable angina? *Eur Heart J* 2000; **21** (**Supplement**): 245.

73. Cominacini L, Fratta Pasini A, Garbin U. Elevated levels of sE-Selectin in patients with IDDM and NIDDM: relation to metabolic control. *Diabetologia* 1995; **38**: 1122–4.

74. Wallen NH, Held C, Rehnqvist N *et al.* Elevated sICAM-1 and sVCAM-1 among patients with stable angina pectoris who suffer cardio-vascular death or non-fatal myocardial infarction. *Eur Heart J* 1999; **14**: 1039–43.

75. Mulvihill N, Foley JB, Murphy RT *et al.* Evidence of sustained inflammation in patients with acute coronary syndromes. *J Am Coll Cardiol* 2000; **36**: 1210–16.

Cardiac metabolism

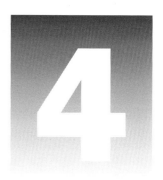

Michael J. Walsh

Physiology of cells

Cell component turnover and cell replication are controlled by genetic programming, and cells can adapt in response to physiological or pathological stimuli.[1] As we get older we tend to lose myocardial cells, and abnormalities of mitochondrial DNA increase with age. It is important to remember that myocardial cells cannot be replicated, and once they have been irreversibly damaged they are lost forever.

Maintenance of the normal structure and function of the heart and blood vessels is based on gene expression directing cellular function. Individual components of the cells, such as ion channels, receptors and enzymes, are continuously renewed. When functional conditions change, gene expression changes to meet the new demands of the cell. The adaptation of the heart and blood vessels to new physiological stimuli and pathological states is regulated by changes in the expression of the genes involved. The function of the cells in the heart and blood vessels depends on a signalling process in which agonists bind to specific receptors on cell surfaces. The signal is then transduced in the cell membrane and within the cell itself by regulatory proteins and second messengers. The term 'receptor' refers to a protein molecule or molecular complex that is capable of recognizing and binding specific transmitter substances and that, as a direct result of such binding, produces a specific biological effect.

The viability of many cells is dependent on a constant or intermittent supply of cytokines or growth factors. In the absence of appropriate cytokine stimulation, cells may undergo programmed cell death (apoptosis). They may also die after overwhelming external injury (necrosis) with accompanying inflammation.

Biology of the vessel wall

The components of the vascular tree are developed in such a way as to allow flexibility of pressure at different parts of the circulation.[1] Major arteries such as the aorta and other elastic vessels expand during systole to accommodate flow. Muscular arteries can vary their calibre in proportion to flow. The resistant arterioles can regulate organ blood flow and vary systemic pressure. Capillaries are 'distributors' of adequate blood flow to body tissues. The veins and venules allow blood to return to the heart under low filling pressure. The endothelial lining of blood vessels has a dynamic function, with specific metabolic, trophic and paracrine functions.

Functions of endothelial cells

Vasomotor tone is to a considerable extent under the control of endothelial cells, which produce several compounds that affect the function of smooth muscle cells, including the following:[1]

1. endothelium-derived relaxing factor (EDRF);
2. prostacycline I_2 (PGI_2);
3. endothelin.

   EDRF, also known as nitrous oxide (NO), is released in response both to a large number of agonists and to pulsatile stretching causing vasodilatation. PGI_2 acts as a powerful vasodilator. Endothelin is the most powerful vasoconstrictor known, and it counteracts the effects of NO and PGI_2. In the physiological state the endothelium produces and binds anticoagulants and prevents thrombosis. A dynamic combination of prevention of platelet adhesion and activation of thrombolytic pathways prevents the formation and growth of thrombi on normal endothelium. Damage to the endothelium interferes with these beneficial properties, and the response of the wall to injury is vasoconstriction and thrombus formation. In addition, inflammatory and immune cytokines can produce changes in endothelial function. It can thus be seen that damage to the wall of a coronary artery (e.g. by angioplasty) may lead to acute responses such as thrombosis and, in addition, proliferation of smooth muscle cells which, in the context of angioplasty, may result in restenosis.

Biology of the myocardial cell

The myocardium is composed of cardiac myocytes, which are tethered within an extracellular scaffolding of fibrillar collagen.[2] Myocytes represent about

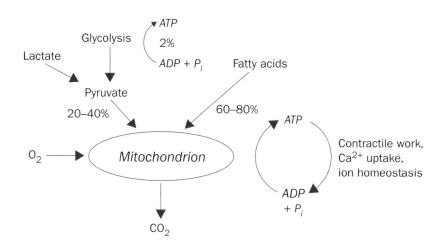

Figure 4.1
Myocardial energy metabolism under aerobic conditions.

one-third of all the cells in the myocardium. Other cells include endothelial and vascular smooth muscle cells of the intramural circulation and fibroblasts located in interstitial and perivascular spaces.

In conditions of normal oxygenation, the metabolism of the heart is governed by the consumption of two major substrates, namely glucose and free fatty acids (see Figure 4.1). The free fatty acid pathway requires more oxygen than the glycolytic pathway to produce an equivalent amount of ATP. Under normal conditions an equilibrium exists between the glucose and free fatty acid pathways, and there is adequate consumption of each energy substrate without metabolic disorder. Myocardial ischaemia is a metabolic event that results from an imbalance between the demands of myocardial cells and myocardial perfusion.

During ischaemia, part of the myocardium becomes anaerobic and the balance of substrates is disturbed, with unoxidized free fatty acid products accumulating (see Figure 4.2). This may result in a reduction in ATP production, a decrease in contractile work and damage to the cell membrane. The inhibition of carbohydrate oxidation causes myocardial contractile dysfunction due to calcium overload, with the accumulation of lactate and hydrogen ions, and consequent acidosis in the cell.[3]

Oxygen extraction from coronary blood is near maximum during basal conditions, so increased extraction represents a very limited source of additional oxygen.[4]

An increase in coronary flow is an effective way of promoting ATP synthesis to match the metabolic needs of the heart. However, when oxygen delivery is interrupted due to coronary artery disease, the balance between ATP production and consumption is disturbed, leading to myocardial ischaemia. In the experimental situation, episodes of coronary arterial occlusion followed by a period of reperfusion and longer episodes of ischaemia

Figure 4.2
Mycocardial energy
metabolism under
anaerobic conditions.

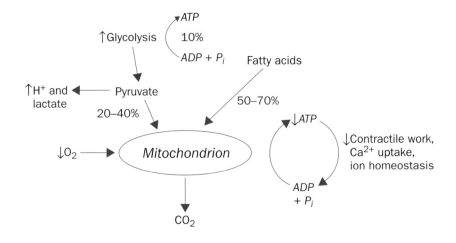

Figure 4.3
Chronology of ischaemia.

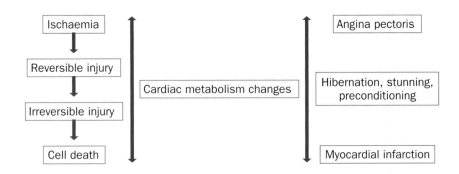

can, in fact, result in some degree of myocardial protection. This is usually termed ischaemic preconditioning.[5]

Occlusion of a major coronary artery in dogs induces injury that is reversible for the first 15 to 20 min, in that complete tissue recovery and serious injury are avoided after reperfusion. However, if the occlusion is maintained beyond this time, the injury becomes irreversible, and some cells die despite reperfusion (see Figure 4.3).

Ischaemic cell death begins in the sub-endocardial region and then progresses with time towards the sub-epicardium. In preconditioned animals, protection is afforded from total occlusion for up to 40 min, but not at 3 h post occlusion. It is suggested that the multiple anginal episodes which often precede myocardial infarction in humans may delay cell death via this mechanism, and that a similar response may occur in patients with unstable angina pectoris. This may allow a greater time window for myocardial salvage through interventions such as angioplasty. There is a possibility that such preconditioning may be a feature in patients who seem to show a 'warm-up' phenomenon with lessening of the angina as exercise continues. However, if the ischaemia continues it will eventually lead to irreversible injury and cell death.

The best technique for assessing metabolic abnormalities of heart muscle cells in humans with ischaemia is positron emission tomography (PET). This technique can be used to study glucose, fatty acid and oxidative metabolism of heart muscle. It is also the best method of assessing myocardial viability.

Stunning

Stunning of the myocardium is a term used to describe reversible mechanical dysfunction that persists despite restoration of normal coronary flow. The condition was first described in 1975,[6] in the experimental situation, with conscious dogs undergoing brief coronary occlusion with reperfusion. There is still much controversy over the role of the actual reperfusion in causing the stunning. The original experiments have been repeated many times and have shown that brief periods of ischaemia (10–15 min) result in a transient delay in functional recovery after restoration of flow. However, the dysfunctional region will recover within hours to days. Hibernation, on the other hand, refers to an ischaemic abnormality due to a severe reduction in coronary flow, which may last for months or years, and which will not recover until the tissue is revascularized.

Stunning and hibernation may of course coexist. In the experimental situation, the stunned myocardium will respond to infusion of inotropic agents such as dobutamine and noradrenaline. Stunning is therefore a relatively mild sub-lethal injury. The debate continues with regard to the pathophysiological mechanisms that result in stunning. Oxygen-derived free radicals such as superoxide, hydrogen peroxide and hydroxyl radicals certainly seem to play a role in the experimental situation. Oxygen-derived free radicals depress myocardial contractility *in vitro* and *in vivo,* but the precise mechanism of this action is not known. The free radicals involved are reactive species that have no specific targets and can attack virtually all cellular components. They can denature proteins and inactivate enzymes, damaging cellular membranes and interfering with the function of the myocardial cell. The free-radical damage is thought to occur early in the reperfusion process.

Abnormalities of calcium homeostasis certainly occur in the ischaemic myocardium, and there is evidence that transient calcium overload during reperfusion may well contribute to the pathogenesis of stunning. However, despite the calcium overload, there is a lack of responsiveness of the myofilaments, as well as a decrease in calcium sensitivity. Inotropic agents can stimulate the stunned myocardium, which suggests that the latter does have a reserve contractile capability, which may be of importance clinically. Clinical situations in which there is transient focal or partial ischaemia followed by early reperfusion include coronary artery spasm, unstable angina, exercise-induced angina, acute myocardial infarction with early reperfusion, coronary angioplasty, coronary artery bypass grafting and valve surgery requiring cardioplegic arrest, and cardiac transplantation. A continuation of the process or recruitment of the stunned areas may be very important in these situations.

It is likely that multiple mechanisms contribute to the pathogenesis of myocardial stunning.[7–9] Stunning interferes with both systolic and diastolic function. It has been shown that wall motion abnormalities in patients with exercise-induced ischaemia can persist for up to 30 min after cessation of exercise.[10] In addition to the contractile abnormalities, exercise induces prolonged metabolic abnormalities, which have been demonstrated using PET. The clinical relevance of this exercise-induced abnormality, which will disappear after exercise, requires further elucidation.

Hibernation

The term 'hibernating myocardium' was introduced by Rahimtoola in the 1980s to describe a state of persistent impairment of resting ventricular dysfunction caused by severe ischaemia that is partially or completely reversible upon restoration of adequate flow.[11] It can be considered to be an adaptive response to a reduction in flow, allowing the myocardium to match its oxygen supply to oxygen demand. Surgeons had known for a long time that sections of the myocardium which were dyskinetic or akinetic prior to operation showed improved function after revascularization. Histologically there is a loss of contractile proteins and cardiac myocytes with loss of cell volume, changes in the cell nucleus and loss of sarcoplasmic reticulum. To some extent the hibernating myocytes regress to an embryonic type.[12] PET has been used to detect hibernating segments of the myocardium and to study the pathophysiology of the adaptive mechanism. It would seem that the hibernating myocardium switches from aerobic to anaerobic metabolism, and that when this occurs the myocardial segments which are involved recover function after revascularization. However, the time-course of recovery after revascularization can be quite variable. Instinctively one would feel that the longer the ischaemia, the slower the subsequent recovery would be. The concept of the hibernating myocardium is interesting in that it emerged from clinical studies and has proved very difficult to study at the basic laboratory level, whereas concepts of stunning and preconditioning emerged from laboratory experimentation. However, if hibernation is a truly adaptive process in relation to ischaemia, then it has immense potential as a mechanism for protecting the myocardium, reducing dysfunction and preventing the onset of heart failure.

Preconditioning

The fact that short periods of ischaemia plus reperfusion in the experimental situation reduce the degree of myocardial damage (infarction) after eventual total occlusion was first demonstrated in 1986.[5] The authors suggested that the multiple anginal episodes that often precede a myocardial infarction in humans may delay cell death after coronary occlusion, and allow a greater time window for intervention to restore flow and prevent myocyte death. Preconditioning is an acute adaptive phenomenon whereby the myocardium reacts to stress in such a way that it is transiently better able to tolerate the stress of subsequent episodes of ischaemia.[12] It has been shown in laboratory experiments that there is a reduction of anaerobic glycolysis with decreased lactate production in the preconditioned state. In addition, much less glycogen is used. Since lactate usually accumulates with ischaemia in myocardium that is not preconditioned, there is therefore less acidosis in the preconditioned myocardium. There is a slowing of the decline in available ATP during ischaemia and reduced energy demand, which is a characteristic feature of preconditioning. The concept of preconditioning raises issues with regard to the occurrence of apoptosis and necrosis in the ischaemic myocardium:

- stunning – normal flow, depressed function;
- hibernation – depressed flow, depressed function;
- preconditioning – repetitive ischaemia may induce tolerance.

Myocardial cell death

Apoptosis, or programmed cell death, is a genetically determined form of cell death that often serves as an essential component of normal postnatal morphogenesis in the human heart.[13] It can also be triggered by noxious stimuli or become uncontrolled after having begun normally, and may then have pathological consequences. *In vitro*, apoptotic changes may occur within seconds or minutes, and cytological characteristics *in vitro* include shrinkage of cell size, clumping and cleaving of the nucleus, early disappearance of the nucleolus and generally a morphological preservation of intracellular organelles such as mitochondria or sarcoplasmic reticulum, and preservation of an intact plasmalemma.[13] Apoptotic cells are eventually phagocytosed. If phagocytic capacities are exceeded, the apoptotic bodies gather in pools but do not damage the surrounding cells. Apoptosis is an orderly process. Necrosis, in contrast, is a disorderly process in which the cells increase in size, the mitochondria and sarcoplasmic reticulum quickly disintegrate, the nucleus deteriorates non-specifically and the plasma membrane ruptures to release all of the intracellular contents into the interstitial space. This is harmful to local cells, with the accumulation of neutrophils and lymphocytes. Haemorrhage into the necrotic area may occur, and areas of liquefaction necrosis may become evident. This does not occur in apoptosis. The relationship between apoptosis and necrosis in ischaemic areas of myocardium has not been elucidated. It has been suggested that stimulation of sensory nerve endings in the heart by acidosis is the initiating event for the pain of angina pectoris, but as this does not occur in apoptotic areas, this might account for the silent ischaemic changes that are seen in patients with angina or myocardial infarction.[13]

In conclusion, the myocyte has specific characteristics which contribute to a unique myocardial physiology. The past two decades have seen great advances in our understanding of concepts such as myocardial hibernation, stunning and preconditioning, but much work has still to be done to elucidate these conditions and turn them to therapeutic advantage.

Acknowledgement

We would like to thank Servier Laboratories for allowing us to use Figures 4.1, 4.2 and 4.3.

References

1. Maseri A. *Ischaemic heart disease. A rational basis for clinical practice and clinical research.* New York: Churchill Livingstone, 1999.
2. Weber KT. Targeting pathological remodeling. Concepts of cardioprotection and reparation. *Circulation* 2000; **102**: 1342–5.
3. Boucher FR, Hearse DJ, Opie LH. Effects of trimetazidine on ischaemic contracture in isolated perfused rat hearts. *J Cardiovasc Pharmacol* 1994; **24**: 45–9.
4. Zarco P, Zarco MH. Biochemical aspects of cardioprotection. *Medicographia* 1996; **18**: 18–21.
5. Murray CE, Jennings RB, Reimer KA. Preconditioning with ischaemia: a delay of lethal cell injury in ischaemic myocardium. *Circulation* 1986; **74**: 1124–36.
6. Heyndrickx GR, Millard RW, McRitchie RJ, Maroko PR, Vatner SF. Regional myocardial functional and electrophysiological alterations after brief coronary artery occlusion in conscious dogs. *J Clin Invest* 1975; **56**: 978–85.
7. Bolli R. Mechanism of myocardial 'stunning'. *Circulation* 1990; **82**: 723–38.

8. Hearse DJ. Stunning: a radical review. *Cardiovasc Drugs Ther* 1991; **5**: 853–76.

9. Ferrari R, La Canna G, Giubbini R *et al.* Left ventricular dysfunction due to stunning and hibernation in patients. *Cardiovasc Drugs Ther* 1994; **8**: 371–80.

10. Robertson WS, Feigenbaum H, Armstrong WF *et al.* Exercise echocardiography: a clinically practical addition in the evaluation of coronary artery disease. *J Am Coll Cardiol* 1983; **2**: 1085–91.

11. Wijns W, Vatner SF, Camici PG. Hibernating myocardium. *N Engl J Med* 1998; **339**: 173–81.

12. Murray CE, Jennings RB, Reimer KA. Preconditioning with ischaemia: a delay of lethal cell injury in ischaemic myocardium. *Circulation* 1986; **74**: 1124–36.

13. James TN. Homage to James B Herrick: a contemporary look at myocardial infarction and at sickle-cell heart disease. The 32nd Annual Herrick Lecture of the Council on Clinical Cardiology of the American Heart Association. *Circulation* 2000; **101**: 1874–87.

Clinical diagnosis

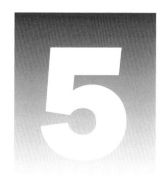

Gerard Gearty

Angina pectoris: the doctor's dilemma

The recurrent chest discomfort, aches, pains and pressures of middle age are, for the majority of humanity, a relatively benign nuisance. However, for a significant minority these symptoms represent the first signs of significant coronary artery disease – a potentially life-threatening condition. Since clinical examination is often normal, the important decision to investigate further depends almost entirely on the patient's symptoms and the overall likelihood of heart disease. As always in the delicate interplay of doctor and patient, one lets the story emerge in the patient's own words with as little direct questioning as possible initially. Subsequently it is important to probe the patient gently along more precise lines to encourage the emergence of a convincing diagnostic pattern. Such a clear pattern is often found in the presence of angina pectoris. Typical angina in the clinical sense consists of effort-related chest discomfort of relatively brief duration, with fairly rapid resolution on resting. This classic pattern is rarely found in any other condition.

Who develops angina? The typical story is of a middle-aged man who is obese, physically unfit and a long-standing smoker, with a positive family history – a high-risk combination. Similar factors, of course, hold true for the female patient, although symptoms emerge on average one decade later. The presence of established diabetes mellitus, hypertension or myxoedema is particularly important. However, this focus on the classic patient can be seriously misleading, since many angina patients exhibit none of these leading signs, and premature heart disease in the younger patient can be overlooked, particularly in women. There is good evidence that female patients have more atypical signs, fewer investigations and a longer wait before diagnosis than their male counterparts.

The history

A clinical analysis of chest pain requires careful consideration of the following:

1. characteristics and intensity;
2. site and radiation;
3. provoking and relieving factors;
4. associated symptoms;
5. the effects of medication – nitrate response.

CHARACTERISTICS AND INTENSITY

Patients will often deny the experience of actual pain, and more often describe a vague diffuse discomfort, pressure or tightness, or sometimes just a rawness or dryness in the throat or indigestion in the chest. Since the pain can be of relatively mild intensity, short duration and transient in nature, there is often a delay of many weeks or months before the first medical consultation. Short, sharp, unprovoked darts or stabs of pain in the chest, left chest cramp or a persistent dull left sub-mammary ache without a consistent relationship to exertion rarely reflect ischaemic pain.

SITE AND RADIATION

The discomfort is usually diffuse and located in the centre of the chest. With increasing intensity it spreads to the root of the neck, the lower jaws, across the shoulders and down the inner arms, particularly on the left side, often with a focus around the elbow or wrist. The common embryological origins of these areas and their shared dermatomal roots explain how difficult it can be to localize a deep visceral pain such as ischaemia. Sometimes angina radiates to the upper back, but rarely to the back of the neck or above the lower jaw. Radiation is of some importance, since atypical anginal syndromes may also present peripherally with ache in the neck or lower jaw, discomfort in the epigastrium, or wrist pain.

PROVOKING AND RELIEVING FACTORS

The presenting discomfort is often exercise provoked, and may be accentuated after meals or in a cold environment. Pain while walking against a cold wind is a classic early warning symptom. Initially, when the condition is relatively mild, it may be possible to walk through this angina, and indeed some patients describe a 'warming up' phenomenon. However, as the disease progresses, pain forces a rapid reduction or cessation of regular exercise. Rest is typically followed by complete resolution of the pain within a couple of minutes. Thus irrespective of the nature of the discomfort, which can be described in so many different ways and at so many different sites, the consistent association with exercise and the equally consistent dramatic relief obtained with rest are strong diagnostic features which rarely occur in any of the other myriad causes of recurring chest discomfort.

ASSOCIATED SYMPTOMS

Anginal pain or pressure may be accompanied by a disconcerting anxiety, distinct dyspnoea or a feeling of weakness that is rather out of proportion to the intensity of any actual pain. A feeling of impending doom, or 'angor animi', is a classic warning symptom. Occasionally the clinical syndrome may be dominated by such symptoms without actual chest pressure, particularly in the diabetic or older patient. Such symptoms may force cessation of activity, and this is characteristically followed by rapid relief. Sometimes the gastrointestinal aspect dominates, with epigastric discomfort associated with a flatulent dyspepsia, which bizzarely can bring relief. Thus indigestion may be the presenting symptom. This impression may be reinforced by a relationship with effort after heavy meals.

THE EFFECTS OF MEDICATION – NITRATE RESPONSE

Nitrate response to a tablet or spray often clears the chest discomfort within 2 to 3 min. However, a nitrate response, although useful, is not specific and can also relax oesophageal spasm. Benefit from the prophylactic use of nitrate is perhaps more convincing evidence of underlying ischaemia.

The clinical examination

What are the clinical findings in the patient with angina pectoris? Often the initial examination is entirely normal. High lipid levels may be suggested by premature corneal arcus, xanthelasma and tendon xanthomata. Blood pressure readings are important, since long-standing systemic hypertension may present for the first time, with persistent pressure readings greater than 140/90 mmHg. Clues to significant arteriopathy may be found by careful clinical examination elsewhere (retinoscopy, carotid bruits, a palpable pulsatile abdominal aorta, diminution or absence of femoral or peripheral arterial pulses).

Auscultation of the heart usually reveals clear normal heart sounds without extra sounds or heart murmurs. Auscultation during pain may occasionally reveal transient extra heart sounds during ischaemia (a gallop rhythm and the soft apical systolic murmur of functional mitral incompetence). Occasionally, anginal discomfort may be the first presentation of significant aortic stenosis indicated by a loud ejection aortic systolic murmur radiating to the root of the neck. Rarely, auscultatory findings may indicate the possibility of sub-aortic stenosis, hypertrophic obstructive cardiomyopathy (HOCM), severe mitral stenosis or pulmonary hypertension, all of which are associated with varying degrees of atypical pain.

Differential diagnosis

It is an important clinical axiom that there are always alternative explanations for pain, no matter how 'classic' the presentation may be at first glance (see Table 5.1). If the clinical picture is incomplete, atypical or unusual in some way, or if the disease does not develop as expected, the possibility arises that the original working diagnosis was wrong or at least incomplete. Recurring musculoskeletal chest pains and aches are very common and usually benign, although for many patients they represent a major and frustrating problem, since management and medication are so often disappointing.

It is important to consider the following:

1. musculoskeletal chest wall pain;
2. anxiety neurosis;
3. angina with normal coronary arteries;
4. gastrointestinal problems;
5. chronic pulmonary problems.

MUSCULOSKELETAL CHEST WALL PAIN

Musculoskeletal chest wall pains and aches are usually focal rather than diffuse. Sharp stabs and darts of pain are common complaints, and persistent

Table 5.1
Differential diagnosis for patients with chest pain

Cardiovascular	Gastrointestinal	Chest wall	Pulmonary	Psychiatric
Pericarditis	Oesophageal	Costochondritis	Asthma	Anxiety
Aortic dissection	Peptic ulcer	Herpes zoster	Pulmonary embolism	Depression
Angina	Reflux	Rib fracture	Pneumonia	Panic disorder
	Biliary colic	Fibrositis	Pleuritis	
	Pancreatitis		Pneumothorax	

ache may also occur in the left sub-mammary area or left subscapular area, persisting for many hours, with no identifiable exertional component. The chest wall may exhibit vague deep tenderness, and local anaesthetic infiltration can sometimes help. Tietze's syndrome,[1] or costochondritis, is firmly enshrined in the literature although it is extremely rare (I am still waiting to see my first case). Patients with musculoskeletal pain occasionally present to the accident and emergency department following a particularly severe cramp in the chest with associated dyspnoea. This type of presentation can mimic an acute coronary syndrome and demands appropriate investigation. Such patients may experience disproportionate effort dyspnoea and often report chronic fatigue, irritable bowel symptoms and long-standing headaches. The causes of these symptoms may lie in social circumstance, and intelligent management of such problems can avoid the need for lengthy and expensive investigations. If symptoms increase in frequency and severity, with effort-related central chest pressure, the clinician may be forced to investigate them more thoroughly.

ANXIETY NEUROSIS

Recurring chest pains, effort dyspnoea, palpitations, extreme fatigue, anxiety and eventual collapse are not problems peculiar to the modern age, and they were a major problem in the armies of yester-year ('soldier's heart'). The best specialist minds of those times failed to identify any tangible disease, and after a convalescent regime with rehabilitation, many of these patients were able to resume their occupation after 6 months. Thomas Lewis described this as 'effort syndrome with strong neurotic basis'. Subsequently he found such symptoms to be common in routine hospital practice.[2] These types of presentations were extensively addressed by Paul Wood and Paul Dudley White in the first half of the last century,[3] both of whom emphasized the chronic but essentially benign nature of the condition, the lack of objective evidence of heart disease, the good prognosis but the considerable morbidity associated with the problem, which was unresponsive to a wide range of management approaches and medication. Unfortunately, perhaps, both authorities dismissed such patients as essentially neurotic, and little was done to advance management of the underlying disorder. It is an important historical lesson that yesterday's orthodoxies may become tomorrow's heresies, and when reading the work of these major authorities of the early twentieth century, there is much to remind one of current controversies about syndrome X and the emerging study of microvascular ischaemia. The psychiatric aspects of non-cardiac chest pain have been usefully reviewed by Chambers *et al.*[4] They discuss the psychological variables and outline the occasional value of antidepressant drugs and cognitive–behavioural therapy.

ANGINA WITH NORMAL CORONARY ARTERIES

Much attention has been focused on microvascular dysfunction – the behaviour of the smaller coronary vessels, which are not adequately visualized at routine angiography. It is suggested that an exaggerated response to vasoconstrictor stimuli and reduced vasodilator reserve and/or abnormal pain perception are important factors. However, findings are inconsistent and therapeutic strategies have so far been disappointing. Syndrome X refers to a specific triad of typical chest pain, typical electrocardiogram (ECG) changes at stress testing, and normal vessels at angiography. Despite abnormalities in flow reserve, perfusion scans and vasomotor endothelial responses, such a syndrome is still associated with an excellent prognosis, and little has been achieved in terms of reliable treatment for the long-suffering patient.

GASTROINTESTINAL PROBLEMS

Oesophageal spasm can cause central chest pressure, with a similar ability to radiate to sites associated with angina, such as the left arm. More confusingly, such spasm may occasionally be relieved by short-acting nitrates. Motility disorders and acid reflux (often provoked by specific dietary irritants) are amenable to dietary manipulation, simple antacids or proton-pump inhibition. Some patients require specialist gastroenterological investigations and oesophageal mobility and pressure studies.

CHRONIC PULMONARY PROBLEMS

Chronic lung disease, recurring bronchial asthma or chronic diffuse lung disease with poor function will cause effort dyspnoea, sometimes associated with unpleasant pressure similar to angina. These smoking-related conditions often coexist with ischaemia, so extreme care must be taken to elicit changes in symptoms over time in these patients.

Summary

There are few serious alternatives to the diagnosis of angina pectoris, once a carefully taken history has elicited a story of chest pain that is brought on by exertion and relieved by rest. The immediate challenge then is to define risk status and plan further investigations to indicate the extent, severity and potential threat implicit in this highly significant diagnosis. For the non-cardiac chest pains, in the context of an ever better educated and motivated public, merely giving reassurance that such discomfort is not cardiac is now inadequate, since physical and psychiatric aspects and possible gastrointestinal problems are often amenable to further definition and intelligent management.

References

1. Braunwald E. *Heart disease: a textbook of cardiovascular medicine*, 5th edn. Philadelphia, PA: W.B. Saunders, 1997.
2. Lewis T. *The soldier's heart and the effort syndrome*, 2nd edn. London: Shaw and Sons, 1940.
3. Wood P. Da Costa's syndrome or effort syndrome. *Br Med J* 1941; **i**: 767, 805, 845.
4. Chambers J, Bass C, Mayou R. Non-cardiac chest pain: assessment and management. *Heart* 1999; **82**: 656–7.

The management of chest pain in general practice

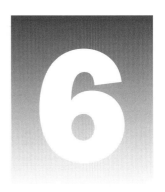

Andrew W. Murphy

Introduction

The objectives of this chapter are first to outline the optimal management of chest pain in general practice, and second to describe, for angina pectoris, the implications of guideline implementation. The latter is especially important, as there are some discrepancies between what the guidelines suggest and current practice. Finally, there will be a brief discussion of the general management of chronic disease in general practice.

This chapter refers only to patients with chronic stable angina. The chapter has been explicitly based on the following specific sources:

- the revised guidelines of the British Cardiac Society and the Royal College of Physicians of London;[1]
- the North of England Evidence-Based Guidelines;[2]
- the recommendations of the Task Force of the European Society of Cardiology;[3]
- the guidelines of the American College of Cardiology/American Heart Association.[4]

A literature search was also performed (see Box 6.1). Where specific recommendations have been made, the categorization system of the North of England Evidence-Based Guidelines[2] has been explicitly utilized unless otherwise stated (see Box 6.2).

Definitions

When patients complain of chest pain, it is the often difficult task of general practitioners to attempt to generate a medical diagnosis. The term

---

Box 6.1   Literature search

The following seven separate literature searches were performed on PubMed in November 2000:

1. angina pectoris [majr] OR chest pain [majr]
   AND
   general practitioner* OR family physician* OR general practice* OR family practice* OR physicians, family*

2. angina pectoris [majr] OR chest pain [majr]
   AND
   incidence [ti] OR incidence [mesh]
   limited to publication date 1995 or later

3. angina pectoris [majr] OR chest pain [majr]
   AND
   (sensitivity and specificity [MESH] OR (predictive [WORD] AND value* [WORD])) limited to REVIEW

4. angina pectoris [majr] OR chest pain [majr]
   AND
   therapy OR treatment OR management
   limited to PRACTICE GUIDELINE

5. angina pectoris [majr] OR chest pain [majr]
   AND
   risk factors
   limited to (REVIEW or META-ANALYSIS) and publication date 1995 or later

6. angina pectoris [majr] OR chest pain [majr]
   AND
   (prognosis [MH:NOEXP] OR survival analysis [MH:NOEXP])
   limited to REVIEW

7. open access
   AND
   ECG OR electrocardiography

---

angina pectoris is reserved for chest discomfort that is considered to be due to myocardial ischaemia associated with coronary artery disease.[3] Two rare additional causes of classical angina, namely aortic stenosis and hypertrophic cardiomyopathy, are referred to. How frequently these are encountered by the general practitioner has not been established. Stable angina refers to symptoms that have been occurring over a period of several weeks without major deterioration. It is important to note that in stable angina, symptoms may also vary considerably from one time to another. Angina is considered

Box 6.2   The categorization system of the North of England Evidence-Based Guidelines (2000)[2]

Category	Type of evidence
I	Evidence from meta-analysis of randomized controlled trials or from at least one randomized controlled trial
II	Evidence from at least one controlled study without randomization or at least one other type of quasi-experimental study
III	Evidence from non-experimental descriptive studies, such as comparative, correlation and/or case–control studies
IV	Evidence from expert committee reports or opinions and/or clinical experience with respected authorities
A	Directly based on category I evidence
B	Directly based on category II evidence or extrapolated recommendation from category I evidence
C	Directly based on category III evidence or extrapolated recommendation from category I or II evidence
D	Directly based on category IV evidence or extrapolated recommendation from category I, II or III evidence

to be unstable if the symptoms worsen abruptly for no apparent reason, if relatively low workloads cause angina, or if it occurs at rest.

Incidence and prevalence in general practice

The community epidemiology of angina was reviewed in Chapter 2 (p. 5). Here we shall discuss those studies that have reviewed general practice incidence and prevalence. The distinction is important, as general practice-based research will obviously reflect the volume and type of work that is currently being identified by existing systems of health care.

Determination of incidence is not just of semantic interest. The implementation of strategies to improve community management of angina will depend crucially on workload, which can only be calculated using accurate incidence and prevalence figures. The North of England Evidence-Based

Table 6.1
Incidence and prevalence general practice studies of angina

Study (year)	Location	Number of practices	Identification method	Number of identified patients (age range in years)	Prevalence (%)	Annual incidence (per 1000 patients)
Fry (1976)[5]	London	1	Prospective (25 years)	268 (over 40)		5
Shaper et al. (1984)[6]	UK	24	Questionnaire and ECG	607 (40–59)[a]	7.9	
Cannon et al. (1998)[7]	Nottingham		Nitrate prescriptions	6856 (all)	1.5	
Smith et al. (1990)[8]	Scotland		Questionnaire and ECG	10,359 (40–59)	5.5 (male) 3.9 (female)[b]	
McCormick et al. (1991)[9]	England and Wales	60	Software transfer		1.14	0.52
Gandhi et al. (1995)[10]	Southampton	17	Prospective (21 months)	110 (31–70)		0.83
Bottomley (1997)[11]	Wakefield	21	Nitrate prescriptions	5131 (all)	3.1	
Gill et al. (1999)[12]	Oxford	1	Record review	146 (45–74)	7.4	9.7
Meale et al. (2000)[13]	Trent	5	Software search	348 (all)	2.25	0.16

[a]Male patients only.
[b]Based on past medical history.

Guidelines (2000)[2] suggest that the 'average' general practitioner will care for 23 patients with angina, who will each have two to three angina-related visits per year. Table 6.1, which provides a chronological review of work in this area, reveals interesting developments in methodological approaches. All of the studies found that prevalence increased with age and was higher among male patients. Studies that utilized nitrate prescribing had lower prevalence estimates than those which employed questionnaires or record review.

There have been fewer incidence studies. In one study,[10] 117 general practitioners agreed to refer to a chest pain clinic 'all patients presenting for the first time with chest pain which could be stable angina'. The reported incidence of angina was 1.13 for males and 0.53 for females per 1000 patients aged 31–70 years per year. There is a striking discrepancy between the reported incidences of this and other studies[12] (see Table 6.1). Gill argues, in my view convincingly, that studies such as that of Gandhi et al.,[10] which depended on single identification strategies, especially referral to secondary care, will significantly underestimate the prevalence and incidence of angina in general practice. Obviously this work needs to be replicated in a larger number of practices.

There has been relatively little analysis of changes in trends over time. The morbidity national studies of the Royal College of General Practitioners are based on a representative sample, from volunteer practices, of approximately 1% of the population of England and Wales. Comparison of the 1991 report with that of 1981 suggests a 60% increase in the prevalence of angina among males and a 69% increase among females. This contrasts with a decrease of 31% in myocardial infarction rates for both males and females. However, some of these changes, for both angina and myocardial infarction, may be accounted for by differences in disease classification between the two time periods. Meale et al.[13] reported results from a total population of 40 000 over a 5-year period from 1993 to 1997. They found a significant decrease in the incidence of ischaemic heart disease generally (including angina), but an increase in myocardial infarction specifically. These apparently conflicting findings require further study. For the present, the results of the national studies, based on their larger size and superior methodology, can be accepted. This would suggest that the workload associated with the management of angina will increase significantly, and that such an increase will be exacerbated as management becomes more intensive.

Suggested guideline management

DIAGNOSIS

The four classical symptoms of angina (location, relationship to exercise, character and duration) are well known to all medical students. Even if only the first two are present and quite typical, the diagnosis of chronic stable angina is probable.[3] A response to glyceryl trinitrate may occur, but it is not specific. Unfortunately, for many patients the presentation is not so clear-cut, and differential diagnoses of oesophageal reflux, peptic ulcer, gallstones and most commonly musculoskeletal disorders must be considered. The diagnosis is a clinical one based on history and examination, and it is suggested that further investigations are mainly aids to management.[2]

For a significant number of patients, no obvious cause can be established. The work of Frank[14] in Liverpool in 1970 highlighted the strikingly different pathologies responsible for chest pain in general practice and hospital. Musculoskeletal chest pain was by far the commonest cause in the former, and cardiac chest pain in the latter.

MANAGEMENT

Obviously all patients should be considered in the light of their own unique physical, social and psychological circumstances. Indeed, it is generally accepted that the functional status of the patient should guide the spectrum and intensity of management, rather than simply using age criteria.

Investigation

All patients with chronic stable angina should have their *fasting serum lipids* measured (category A). It is often suggested that patients should also have a *full blood count, thyroid function test* and *glucose measurement*. The evidence for this is not apparent (category D). It is also recommended that patients should have a *resting 12-lead ECG* (category B). It is important to note that the main reason for this is to identify those patients who have a poor prognosis, as any abnormality in the ECG suggests a poor prognosis.

A key component in establishing the prognosis is *exercise electrocardiography*. Traditionally, exercise testing has been used for diagnostic purposes. The test has a diagnostic sensitivity of around 70% and a specificity of approximately 90%.[3] The pre-test likelihood of patients having angina will obviously have significant implications for the number of false-positive and false-negative results. False positives are more common in female patients. It has therefore been suggested that the role of exercise testing is to provide information about prognosis and to identify those who would benefit from further (generally invasive) tests.[1,2] All patients with definite angina should have a prognostic exercise test while taking their normal medication (category B).

Although the international guidelines[1,3,4] have complicated and differing algorithms for the diagnosis of angina, all of them agree that exercise testing should be made available to all patients for prognostic purposes. The European guidelines (1997)[3] suggest that for elderly patients with well-controlled mild symptoms, a resting ECG alone will suffice.

'Direct' or 'open' access to stress testing has been shown to be safe, feasible and considered helpful by general practitioners.[15-17] These studies confirmed that a technician-run open-access service was safe and effective. Reductions in the number of referrals to cardiology services of 47%[17] and 50%[16] were also noted. If open-access testing is not available, patients should generally be referred through a cardiologist for such testing (category B).

Risk-marker modification

Patients with established heart disease, such as angina, are the first priority for coronary heart disease prevention in clinical practice.[18] Such patients have an increased absolute 5-year risk of a subsequent vascular event of more than 20%.[19] Furthermore, although they represent about 5% of the population, about half of all coronary heart disease deaths occur in this group.

Cholesterol

It has been suggested that all patients with overt atherosclerotic disease should be started on a statin.[20] The total serum cholesterol concentration should be lowered below 5 mmol/L *or* by 20–25% (or low-density-lipoprotein-cholesterol levels should be lowered to less than 3 mmol/L *or* by 30%), whichever results in the lower concentration.[21] The *British National Formulary* (*BNF*)[22] states that statins are the drugs of first choice for treating hypercholesterolaemia, fibrates are the first choice for treating hypertriglyceridaemia, and statins or fibrates can be used either alone or together to treat mixed hypertriglyceridaemia. Combination therapy obviously increases the incidence of side-effects, including myositis and hepatic dysfunction.

Blood pressure

All patients should have their blood pressure reduced to consistently lower than 140/85 mmHg.[18] An evidence-based approach to the management of hypertension is outlined in the British Hypertension Society guidelines.[23]

Smoking cessation

Patients who are currently smokers should be advised to stop and, if appropriate, helped to do so (category A). Stopping smoking will probably not alter the anginal symptoms, but it will reduce mortality. Support given to patients who wish to stop smoking will generally include brief advice, and the enhanced value of nicotine replacement therapy is well established. It is important to note that transdermal nicotine is safe to use in patients with ischaemic heart disease, although the *BNF* advises[22] that its use should be avoided in patients with severe cardiovascular disease. Bupropion is also of proven efficacy, although its relative effectiveness with regard to nicotine replacement therapy in the general practice setting has yet to be established,[24] and there has been some concern about arrhythmogenicity.

Exercise

Moderate exercise may be recommended (category C), although the evidence regarding its effects on the morbidity or mortality of angina patients is poorly defined. Nevertheless, regular exercise does improve general patient well-being and lipid and blood pressure control.

Weight reduction and diet

Hypertensive patients with stable angina and an elevated body mass index (BMI) should lose weight until their BMI is as close to normal as possible (category A). The evidence for normotensive patients with a raised BMI is equivocal. The role of a 'Mediterranean diet' and twice-weekly consumption of oily fish in patients with angina and no previous myocardial infarction is unclear.

Drug treatment

This is reviewed extensively in Chapter 9 (p. 117). It is reasonable to state a number of key points of particular pertinence to general practice management.

- In secondary prevention, the role of aspirin, 75 mg daily, is well established (category A). For patients who cannot take aspirin, the ADP-receptor antagonist clopidogrel is widely used, and has been shown to have as good, if not better, preventative efficacy as aspirin.
- If attacks occur more than twice a week, regular symptomatic treatment should be considered. There is clinical evidence for the efficacy of beta-blockers, calcium-channel blockers and nitrates in symptom control compared with placebo. There is also a role for trimetazidine (a cellular antioxidant) and nicorandil (the new K^+-channel opener) in this context. There are also certain benefits of combination therapy. However, there is little evidence for the superiority of one class over another in terms of symptom relief. There is no direct evidence that any class has a significant effect on mortality or myocardial infarction incidence in primary prevention.
- Both British[1] and European[3] guidelines suggest that beta-blockers should be used as first-line treatment (category B). The underlying rationale for this is that the use of beta-blockers in patients post myocardial infarction has shown significant reductions in mortality. It is therefore assumed that this can be extended to patients who have not yet suffered a myocardial infarction. In addition, it is well established that patients who are taking beta-blockers and who subsequently have a myocardial infarction have a lower mortality rate. Beta-blockers should not be terminated suddenly;[21] it is reasonable to taper them off over a 4-week period.
- The choice of drug for patients who cannot take beta-blockers is unclear.
- Choosing a second drug is problematic. Tailoring drugs to individual patient profiles is appropriate. The *BNF*[22] recommends beta-blockers,

followed by dihydropyridine calcium-channel blockers and then long-acting nitrates.

- When choosing a third drug, the UK guidelines[1] suggest there is little evidence that the use of three or more anti-anginal agents provides any additional advantage (category D). Such patients should be referred for a cardiological opinion.

Referral to a cardiologist

The indications for referral to a cardiologist are unclear. The North of England Evidence-Based Guidelines (2000)[2] recommend referral for patients (category D):

- with an uncertain diagnosis;
- who are not adequately controlled on full doses of two drugs;
- who are considered appropriate for further prognostic investigation (e.g. patients with high-risk occupations);
- if open-access exercise testing is not available.

Patient review

For uncomplicated patients with established optimal management, an annual review (category D) is a commonsense approach.

Social aspects: driving

The Driving and Vehicle Licencing Agency (DVLA) webpage for the UK government (www.dvla.gov.uk/@_a_glance/ch2_cardiovascular.htm) (accessed on 13 November 2000) specifies that for group 1 entitlement drivers with stable angina, driving should cease if symptoms occur at rest or at the wheel. Driving may recommence when satisfactory symptom control has been achieved, and the DVLA need not be notified. For group 2 entitlement, relicensing is permitted when the driver has been free from angina for at least 6 weeks, provided that the exercise requirements can be met.

Implications of guideline implementation

The guidelines referred to in this chapter do differ somewhat in specific details, but all of them suggest a revised approach and more intensive management of patients with angina in the community. These implications will now be discussed.

PATIENT IDENTIFICATION

The Joint British Angina Guidelines[18] emphasize the role of audit, which in turn depends on accurate identification of suitable patients. Table 6.1

highlights the wide range of angina prevalence found in different practices in different studies. This range may actually be greater, as the problem of generalizability from practices participating in research to the general community is well recognized. Indeed, one report[25] documented wide variation (from 29% to 100%) in practice registration of patients with established heart disease. Patients with a history of myocardial infarction, rather than angina, were more likely to be included in the register. Inclusion on a register was strongly associated with the provision of optimal treatment. Recent research[26] has clarified the role of practice computer coding with and without drug searches in the identification of patients with ischaemic heart disease. The Read code for ischaemic heart disease (G3) or prescribing of nitrate or aspirin had a sensitivity of 89% and a positive predictive value of 46%.

In general practice, angina encompasses a heterogenous group of patients, ranging from those who have been extensively investigated in hospital to some who have been empirically placed on symptomatic treatment, with or without aspirin. This spectrum is often but not necessarily dependent on functional status or age. In contrast, guidelines approach angina as a single entity. This discrepancy requires further consideration.

EXERCISE TESTING AND RAPID ASSESSMENT CHEST PAIN CLINICS

The guidelines concur that exercise testing should be used for prognostic reasons, suggesting that for many patients diagnosis will be solely clinically based. The Joint British Angina Guidelines[1] suggest, in an investigation algorithm, that exercise testing should be reserved for male patients who are able to exercise and who have a normal resting ECG. This is in marked contrast to current practice. For example, the reported proportion of patients who are referred for open-access stress testing in order to determine their prognosis has been in the range 18–20%.[16,17] Many patients had a low prior probability of ischaemic heart disease, making the interpretation of results problematic. Significant numbers of patients who were identified as either being at high prognostic risk[17] or having a 'strongly' positive test[16] did not receive further optimal management. It is unclear whether this was due to patient reluctance to undergo further diagnostic procedures.

Partly in order to overcome these difficulties, 'rapid assessment chest pain clinics' have been established[27] (see Chapter 7, p. 87). The objectives of these clinics are to provide, through the rapid access of cardiology opinion, 'same-day' diagnosis, treatment, management and follow-up. It is claimed that such clinics provide general practitioners with a firm diagnosis for 90% of patients, identify those patients who require further invasive investigation, and safely reassure those who do not. Further guideline detail on patient diagnosis and the relative roles of clinical assessment, stress testing, rapid assessment chest pain clinics and invasive investigations would be welcome. Such detail would include the expected proportions and numbers of patients per practice who were undergoing the different investigations.

MANAGEMENT

There are few data on the proportion of patients with angina who have had full blood counts, thyroid function tests, glucose measurements and resting ECGs. It is reasonable to suggest that such practice is not widespread for all patients. Due to the high prevalence of angina, and its apparently increasing incidence, the workload implications of this more intensive approach are significant. The guidelines could be more explicit about the role of risk stratification in test determination.

Similarly, the use of beta-blockers as first-line agents, the choice of a second drug and the avoidance of third-line agents, unless patient referral has occurred, do not appear to have been reported. Provisional audit reports could presumably be generated using computerized prescribing records. The optimal management of cholesterol levels and blood pressure will certainly involve frequent (at least quarterly) practice visits until these parameters are stabilized. Many practitioners review stabilized patients at least twice a year. The implications for general practice workload are obvious.

Table 6.2 reports the results of intervention studies of the provision of care for patients with established heart disease. The provision of aspirin and management of hypertension according to agreed guidelines are good, with the management of lipids in all studies appearing to be suboptimal. The lipid results from the health survey of England suggest that of all the participants aged 16–75 years, 440 individuals reported a history of coronary heart disease (angina or previous myocardial infarction).[28] Of these, 72% reported having had their cholesterol level measured at least once, with 88% reporting a cholesterol level higher than 5 mmol/L or being on treatment. Based on a single non-fasting study assay, 15% of the male patients and 9% of the female patients with established heart disease had controlled cholesterol levels of less than 5 mmol/L. The study was conducted in 1998, before the publication of more recent guidelines with lower cholesterol levels. Nevertheless, as it is based on a random community sample, rather than participating research practices, the results are noteworthy.

It would be informative for audits to discriminate between the diagnostic groups. It appears reasonable to suggest that patients who have had the most 'dramatic' clinical histories and investigative pathways will be more likely to receive optimal care. Therefore global analyses may mask significant under-provision of care for patients with angina only. The separate analyses in the

Table 6.2
General practice intervention studies of the provision of care for patients with established heart disease
(please refer to footnotes for description of study data)

	Cupples and McKnight		SHIP study[b]		Grampian study[c]		POST study[d]	
Reference	Cupples and McKnight 1994[29]		Jolly et al. 1999[30]		Campbell et al. 1998[31,32]		Feder et al. 1999[34]	
Year of study	1991[a]		1995/96		1996/97		1995/97	
Study location	Belfast		Southampton		Grampian region		Hackney	
Patient population	Working diagnosis of angina in general practices		Hospital recruitment of survivors of myocardial infarction or new angina		Working diagnosis of coronary heart disease in general practice		Hospital recruitment of survivors of myocardial infarction or unstable angina	
Intervention	Personal health education by nurse		Co-ordinated care by liaison nurses		Nurse-run clinics		Postal prompts to patients and GPs	
	Control	Intervention	Control	Intervention	Control	Intervention	Control	Intervention
Total sample	300	317	87	65	630	635	156	172
Mean systolic pressure (mmHg)	136	137	146	136	142			
Mean diastolic pressure (mmHg)	77	77	87	82	81			

Category								
Mean cholesterol concentration (mmol/L)	6.0	6.0	5.9	5.7	6.5	6.5		
Aspirin uptake (%)	76	80	76	80	67	81	91	90
Management of hypertension according to guidelines (%)			94	96	88	97		
Management of lipids according to guidelines (%)			57	62	22	41		
Current smokers (%)	17	16	14	19	15	17		

[a] A 5-year follow-up study of this group is available.[33]

[b] In the SHIP study, at 1-year follow-up there were 267 controls and 235 intervention patients, of whom 87 and 65 subjects, respectively, had a history of angina. Figures for all categories refer to angina patients only. SHIP defined high blood pressure as systolic > 160 mmHg or diastolic > 100 mmHg. Management of lipids according to guidelines refers to patients with 'cholesterol > 5.5 but not receiving treatment'.

[c] In the Grampian study, 45% of patients were reported to have had a previous myocardial infarction, but separate reports by diagnostic category are not available. Figures for mean systolic pressure, mean diastolic pressure and mean cholesterol level refer to baseline data for all respondents ($n = 1343$). Follow-up was at 1 year.

[d] In the POST study, 41% of patients were reported to have an initial diagnosis of unstable angina, but separate reports by diagnostic category are not available. Follow-up was at 6 months. Recorded blood pressure measurements were similar for intervention groups (90%) and control groups (84%). A significantly higher proportion of patients in the intervention group had their serum cholesterol level measured (64% vs. 35%; $P < 0.001$). The proportion who were offered smoking advice was increased among the intervention group (69% vs. 44%; $P < 0.05$).

Southampton Heart Integrated Care Project (SHIP),[30] a study of patients with myocardial infarction or angina, support this view. However, the patient numbers are small and the results are somewhat conflicting. Aspirin use has been found to be lower among patients with angina only compared with those who have a history of myocardial infarction.[31]

All of the studies in Table 6.2 noted the shortcomings of their respective interventions in achieving optimal care for many patients. Bradley *et al.*, in a landmark paper using the SHIP study as a case study,[35] reviewed the interpretation of the results of complex health service interventions. They emphasized the importance of understanding the people with whom, and the context within which, the intervention is operationalized. Guidelines are about generalizable evidence, but their implementation must take into account the local diverse systems of practice organization and the individual and disparate patient approaches to lifestyle changes.

General management of chronic disease

The impact of guidelines on physician behaviour has been generally disappointing. Guidelines which increase practice workload pose particular implementation challenges. There have been calls for fewer and more concise guidelines,[36] for both practitioners and patients, to be available in a variety of forms. Angina guidelines appear to be a suitable case for such treatment.

It is generally accepted that successful chronic disease management in general practice requires good interface communication and a co-ordinated multidisciplinary team (which for angina usually refers to administrative staff, general practitioners and practice nurses). Nurses are usually expected to perform complementary and supplementary functions. It has been shown that practice nurses are enthusiastic about such care, but successful delivery requires appropriate training and support (both structural and moral) from general practitioners.[37] The spectrum of cardiac patients' views about the involvement of practice nurses in their follow-up care is wide.[38] Such views are influenced by the patients' perceptions both of the seriousness of their condition and of the practice organization, specifically the status of practice nurses in the primary care team. The full potential of angina management in general practice will only be realized when such requirements are met.

The National Service Framework for Coronary Heart Disease[21] is intended both to describe and to deliver best care. Standard 3 states that 'general practitioners and primary care teams should identify all people with established cardiovascular disease and offer them comprehensive advice and appropriate treatment to reduce their risks.' Statement 8 notes that 'people with symptoms of angina or suspected angina should receive appropriate investigation and treatment to relieve their pain and reduce their risk of coronary heart events.' Suggested milestones include the establishment of practice-based coronary heart disease registers, with the application of protocols to these patients.

Clear deficiencies of current registers have been identified,[25] and there is bountiful evidence of the incomplete and variable application of evidence in practice. Three essential ingredients are important for such application, namely research, performance measurement and quality improvement.[39] Although, for angina, the detail of the first two ingredients is apparent, the third, namely quality improvement, remains the Holy Grail of general practice research. The knights suggested by the Framework are local, and include Health Improvement Programmes, Long-Term Service Agreements, local networks and clinical governance. This organizational array is impressive, and it is hoped that it will have a significant impact. The workload implications of such programmes on primary care teams and the other work that is daily expected of them are unclear. 'Single disease frameworks' do not rest easily within the comprehensive essence of primary care. How everyday unfiltered, diffuse and tangible patient complaints can be married with the provision of systematic and co-ordinated care will determine the nature and success of attempts to improve the community management of patients with angina.

Summary

Background

- The prevalence of angina is increasing significantly.
- In general practice, angina encompasses a heterogenous group of patients, although the guidelines approach angina as a single entity. This discrepancy requires further consideration.
- Intervention studies on the provision of care have noted shortcomings in achieving optimal care for many patients.

Management

- Diagnosis is clinically based on history and examination, with further investigations mainly functioning as aids to management.
- A key component of establishing the prognosis is exercise electrocardiography. 'Open' access to exercise testing has been shown to be safe and feasible. However, some patients are inappropriately referred, and not all patients who are identified as being at high prognostic risk receive optimal treatment.
- 'Rapid assessment chest pain clinics' have been established to provide a same-day cardiological opinion.

- A clear strategy for dealing with emergency presentations, unstable angina, etc., should be developed according to local facilities and needs.
- The functional status of patients should guide the spectrum and intensity of management.
- If attacks occur more than twice a week, regular symptomatic treatment should be considered. For all the main drug classes for stable angina there is no evidence of relative superiority in terms of mortality or myocardial infarction incidence.
- Patients with established heart disease, such as angina, are the first priority for coronary heart disease prevention.
- All patients with confirmed angina should have their fasting serum lipids measured and a resting 12-lead ECG performed.
- All patients should have their blood pressure reduced to consistently lower than 140/85 mmHg.
- Smokers should be advised to stop and, if appropriate, helped to do so.
- All patients with overt atherosclerotic disease should be started on a statin.
- Hypertensive patients with stable angina and an elevated BMI should lose weight until their BMI is as close to normal as possible.
- Inclusion on a patient register is associated with optimal treatment.
- Practice nurses have a vital role to play in the provision of care for patients with angina.

Acknowledgements

I am grateful to Hugh Brazier for the original search strategy and Edward O'Loghlen for article retrieval. Hugh Brazier and Drs Neil Campbell and Peter Cantillon commented on previous drafts of this chapter.

References

1. de Bono D for the Joint Working Party of the British Cardiac Society and Royal College of Physicians of London. Investigation and management of stable angina: revised guidelines 1998. *Heart* 1998; **81**: 546–55.
2. North of England Evidence-Based Guidelines Development Project. *The primary care management of stable angina.* Newcastle upon Tyne: Centre for Health Services Research, University of Newcastle upon Tyne, 2000.
3. Task Force of the European Society of Cardiology. Management of stable angina pectoris. *Eur Heart J* 1997; **18**: 394–413.
4. American College of Cardiology/American Heart Association. Guidelines for the management of patients with chronic stable angina. *Circulation* 1999; **23**: 2829–48.

5. Fry J. The natural history of angina in a general practice. *J R Coll Gen Pract* 1976; **26**: 643–6.

6. Shaper AG, Cook G, Walker M *et al.* Prevalence of ischaemic heart disease in middle-aged British men. *Br Heart J* 1984; **51**: 595–605.

7. Cannon PJ, Connell PA, Stockley H *et al.* Prevalence of angina as assessed by a survey of prescriptions for nitrates. *Lancet* 1998; **i**: 979–81.

8. Smith WCS, Kenicer MB, Tunstall-Pedoe H *et al.* Prevalence of coronary heart disease in Scotland: Scottish Heart Health Study. *Br Heart J* 1990; **64**: 295–8.

9. McCormick A, Fleming D, Charlton J. *Morbidity statistics in general practice. Fourth national study 1991/92.* Series MB5 No. 3. London: HMSO, 1995.

10. Gandhi MM, Lampe FC, Wood DA. Incidence, clinical characteristics, and short-term prognosis of angina pectoris. *Br Heart J* 1995; **73**: 193–8.

11. Bottomley A. Methodology for assessing the prevalence of angina in primary care using practice-based information in Northern England. *J Epidemiol Commun Health* 1997; **51**: 87–9.

12. Gill D, Mayou R, Dawes M *et al.* Management and course of angina and suspected angina in primary care. *J Psychosom Res* 1999; **46**: 349–58.

13. Meale AG, Pringle M, Hammersley V. Time changes in new cases of ischaemic heart disease in general practice. *Fam Pract* 2000; **17**: 394–400.

14. Frank PI. *Anterior chest pain in general practice.* MD thesis, University of Liverpool, 1970.

15. McClements BM, Campbell NPS, Cochrane D *et al.* Direct-access exercise electrocardiography. *Br Heart J* 1994; **71**: 531–5.

16. Sulke AN, Paul VE, Taylor CJ *et al.* Open-access exercise electrocardiography. *J R Soc Med* 1991; **84**: 590–4.

17. Agrawal S, Danbouchi SS, Goodfellow J *et al.* Technician-run open-access exercise electrocardiography. *Heart* 1999; **82**: 378–82.

18. British Cardiac Society, British Hyperlipidaemia Association, British Hypertension Society and British Diabetic Association. Joint British recommendations on prevention of coronary heart disease in clinical practice: summary. *Br Med J* 2000; **320**: 705–8.

19. Dyslipidaemia Advisory Group. National Heart Foundation clinical guidelines for the assessment and management of dyslipidaemia. *NZ Med J* 1996; **109**: 224–32.

20. Anon. Statin therapy: what now? *Drug Ther Bull* 2001; **39**: 17–19.

21. Department of Health. *Coronary heart disease: National Service Framework*; http://www.doh.gov.uk/nsf/coronary/htm (April 2001).

22. British Medical Association (2000) *British National Formulary.* London: British Medical Association and Royal Pharmaceutical Society of Great Britain, 2000.

23. Ramsay LE, Williams B, Johnston GD *et al.* British Hypertension Society guidelines for hypertension management 1999: summary. *Br Med J* 1999; **319**: 630–5.

24. Anonymous. Bupropion to aid smoking cessation. *Drug Ther Bull* 2000; **38**: 73–5.

25. Moher M, Yudkin P, Turner R, Schofield T, Mant D. An assessment of morbidity registers for coronary heart disease in primary care. *Br J Gen Pract* 2000; **50**: 706–9.

26. Gray J, Majeed A, Kerry S, Rowlands G. Identifying patients with ischaemic heart disease in general practice: cross-sectional study of paper and computerised medical records. *Br Med J* 2000; **321**: 548–50.

27. Newby DE, Fox KAA, Flint LL *et al.* A 'same-day' direct-access chest pain clinic: improved management and reduced hospitalisation. *Q J Med* 1998; **91**: 333–7.

28. Primatesta P, Poulter NR. Lipid concentrations and the use of lipid-lowering drugs: evidence from a national cross-sectional survey. *Br Med J* 2000; **321**: 1322–5.

29. Cupples M, McKnight A. Randomised controlled trial of health promotion in general practice for patients at high cardiovascular risk. *Br Med J* 1994; **309**: 993–6.

30. Jolly K, Bradley F, Sharp S *et al.* for the SHIP Collaborative Study. Randomised controlled trial of follow-up care in general practice of patients with myocardial infarction and angina: final results of the Southampton Heart Integrated Care Project (SHIP). *Br Med J* 1999; **318**: 706–11.

31. Campbell NC, Ritchie LD, Thain J *et al.* Secondary prevention in coronary heart disease: baseline survey of provision in general practice. *Br Med J* 1998; **316**: 1430–4.

32. Campbell NC, Thain J, Deans HG *et al.* Secondary prevention in coronary heart disease: a randomised trial of nurse-led clinics in primary care. *Heart* 1998; **80**: 447–52.

33. Cupples M, McKnight A. Five-year follow-up of patients at high cardio-vascular risk who took part in a randomised controlled trial of health promotion. *Br Med J* 1999; **319**: 687–8.

34. Feder G, Griffiths C, Eldridge S *et al.* Effect of postal prompts to patients and general practitioners on the quality of primary care after a coronary event (POST): randomised controlled trial. *Br Med J* 1999; **318**: 1522–6.

35. Bradley F, Wiles R, Kinmonth A-L *et al.* for the SHIP Collaborative Study. Development and evaluation of complex interventions in health service research: case study of the Southampton Heart Integrated Care Project (SHIP). *Br Med J* 1999; **318**: 712–16.

36. Baker R. Is it time to review the idea of compliance with guidelines? (Editorial). *Br J Gen Pract* 2001; **51**: 107.

37. Wright L, Griffin S, Bradley F. Factors affecting practice nurse involve-ment in follow-up care of patients following myocardial infarction. *Fam Pract* 1998; **15**: 426–30.
38. Wiles R. Empowering practice nurses in the follow-up of patients with established heart disease: lessons from patients' experiences. *J Adv Nurs* 1997; **26**: 729–35.
39. Davis RM, Wagner EG, Groves T. Advances in managing chronic dis-ease. *Br Med J* 2000; **320**: 525–6.

Chest pain assessment units: their role in the emergency department

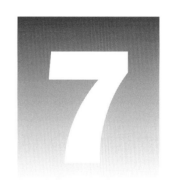

Geraldine McMahon

Introduction and background

Ischaemic heart disease continues to be one of the leading causes of premature death in Western society. The latest World Health Organization figures demonstrate that Ireland, Finland and the UK have the highest mortality from circulatory disease in Europe.[1] There is also a significant degree of morbidity in those who survive acute myocardial infarction, and in those with stable angina. The majority of deaths secondary to acute myocardial infarction occur before the patient reaches hospital.[2] Many of these deaths are potentially preventable by early access to acute medical services. However, much of the evidence suggests that the most cost-effective way to reduce the overall death toll from ischaemic heart disease is through successful implementation of secondary preventative measures.[3]

Chest pain accounts for 2–4% of all new attendances at the emergency department.[4] It is the presenting symptom for a wide variety of medical conditions other than acute coronary syndromes. These range from acute life-threatening conditions such as pulmonary emboli, to minor conditions such as muscle strain. Therefore rapid triage, assessment and management of patients with acute chest pain are an integral part of the routine emergency medicine clinical workload. The traditional approach to the assessment of patients with potential acute coronary syndromes is to evaluate their history,

12-lead electrocardiogram (ECG) and biochemical markers. However, all three aspects of the assessment of this patient group have significant limitations, resulting in inappropriate discharge of high-risk patients and unnecessary admission of others in whom the diagnosis is unclear.

Studies conducted in the UK and the USA show that approximately 12% of patients who present with chest pain are discharged inappropriately from the emergency department.[4] Inappropriate discharge of patients with acute myocardial infarction is associated with a mortality rate of 26%.[5,6] This compares with an inpatient mortality rate of only 6–15%. Younger patients are more likely to be discharged, and are also the group with the highest mortality. Legal costs resulting from inappropriate discharge represent one of the largest sources of litigation in the USA, accounting for 20% of all litigation costs. Clearly there are also significant social and economic costs associated with preventable deaths in this group.

On the other hand, admission of patients with a 'low-risk' profile for serial data is costly in an already over-stretched health service. In a recent study of over 10 000 patients who were admitted from the emergency department following an episode of chest pain, only 17% fulfilled the criteria for acute ischaemia (8% had an acute myocardial infarction (AMI) and 9% had unstable angina).[7] Of the remainder, 6% had stable angina, 21% had other cardiac problems and 55% ultimately had a diagnosis of non-cardiac chest pain. Therefore of all the patients who are formally admitted to hospital with chest pain (? cardiac), over 50% will have no significant cardiac abnormality.

Coronary care units (CCUs) were first developed in the 1960s in order to provide high-intensity medical and nursing care for patients with critical myocardial ischaemia. Admission to CCUs is relatively expensive compared with admission to the general ward, due to the higher ratio of nursing staff to patients and high-intensity monitoring. CCUs have been shown to be highly effective in managing arrhythmia prophylaxis and resuscitation in the early post-myocardial infarction phase.[8–10] Despite the recent advances in rapid assessment systems for acute chest pain in the USA, up to 70% of patients who are admitted to CCUs are there to rule out myocardial infarction.

In the UK, only 61% of admitted patients who are diagnosed with AMI are admitted to CCUs,[11] and conversely as few as 30% of CCU admissions are diagnosed with AMI. This suggests ongoing inconsistencies with regard to the management of acute cardiac presentations.

The chest pain assessment unit

The initial evaluation of patients presenting to the emergency department with symptoms suggestive of AMI is based on the clinical history, physical examination, resting ECG and a single set of cardiac enzymes. However, there is now overwhelming evidence that these assessment tools alone are inadequate.

Over the past few years, systems for the assessment of myocardial ischaemia, which utilize diagnostic tests within the limitations of their maximum clinical utility, have been successfully researched and introduced in order to rationalize the approach to safe and rapid ruling out of AMI. The majority of these units initially focused solely on ruling out AMI. However, many of these units have now extended their role to conducting functional assessments of the myocardium in order to identify patients at high risk of underlying ischaemia.

These assessment units should operate with a low threshold for admission in order to overcome the tendency to discharge patients inappropriately. Patients undergo cardiac marker assessment and computer-assisted ST-segment ischaemia monitoring. In general, this assessment phase can be completed within a period of 6–12 h depending on the protocols used.

A model of this approach was first developed in Amsterdam in 1972. A special unit called 'Eerste Hart Hulp' (cardiac emergency unit) operated a 'precoronary care' type of unit. The main objective at that time was to rationalize admissions to coronary care and to facilitate safe discharge of potential cardiac patients. Similar units were created in other hospitals in The Netherlands. These early 'precoronary care units' provided ECG arrhythmia monitoring, sequential measurements of cardiac markers (creatine kinase (CK), CK-MB) and functional assessments of myocardial perfusion. The introduction of 'precoronary care units' successfully reduced the proportion of patients not at immediate risk who were admitted to CCUs, and facilitated the early discharge of low-risk patients. In the USA, the first chest pain assessment unit was established in the early 1980s by Dr Raymond Bahr, at St Agnes Hospital in Baltimore. Since then, the concept of a rapid cardiac assessment unit for 'low-risk' cardiac-type presentations has continued to be implemented throughout the USA and Europe.

Why is the early assessment of chest pain so difficult?

There are many factors that contribute to the difficulties in early assessment of patients who present with chest pain of cardiac origin. Broadly, they can be divided into doctor-related factors, patient-related factors and factors relating to the limitations of diagnostic tests.

DOCTOR-RELATED FACTORS

There are considerable differences between the health-care systems of the UK and the USA. Emergency care in the USA is predominantly delivered by fully trained emergency care physicians (Attendings). The level of supervision of junior emergency department doctors is considerably higher. In the USA system, all patients are discussed with or seen directly by an Attending prior to discharge.[12] The degree of availability of support from senior colleagues has been identified as an important factor influencing the rate of 'near misses' in patient evaluation.[13] Lack of experience is another factor that has been clearly identified in cases of missed AMI that proceed to litigation. In a study that examined the number of years of experience of doctors who had been successfully sued for the inappropriate discharge of patients with AMI, the experience level was found to be only 2.6 years, compared with 5.1 years of experience in the control group.[13]

Biological variation in the doctor may also contribute to difficulties in performance. Emergency department doctors working a shift pattern may be deprived of sleep or rest, and the stress incurred by a busy department with many sick patients may affect their ability to function effectively. For example, it is known that the mean number of errors in ECG interpretation increases with sleep deprivation.[14] In addition, the necessity for rapid turnover, quick consultation and decision making in a busy and noisy emergency department may put pressure on the doctor to make quick decisions, which may further impair the decision-making process.

PATIENT-RELATED FACTORS

These factors also contribute to difficulties with regard to accurate early assessment. Cardiac disease does not always have a typical presentation. The emergent nature of the disease means that it may not be considered or it may be ruled out due to lack of a classical history and/or diagnostic features, which may not yet have developed fully at the time of evaluation. The characteristics of the chest pain are important. As many as 25% of AMI cases will present with atypical features, and 25% of them may have no symptoms at all (silent AMI).[15] These patients are more likely to be discharged. Such problems have led to specific pathways to deal systematically with chest pain.

THE TRIAGE SYSTEM

'Triage' is a French word meaning 'to sort'. A wide variety of undifferentiated acute medical emergencies can present to the emergency department at any one time. These patients need to be prioritized primarily according to the degree of 'threat to life' that is posed by their condition. The Manchester Triage System is now widely used in the UK. This system involves an assessment of the patients' clinical priority based on their presenting symptoms and a series of general discriminators and specific discriminators. The general discriminators refer to aspects of the assessment that include the overall threat to life (compromised airway, breathing or circulation), the severity of pain, haemorrhage, level of consciousness and temperature. Specific discriminators are those that are specific for a particular symptom complex (e.g. chest pain). Patients who present with chest pain typical of 'cardiac-type' are triaged as 'very urgent', which implies a target time of 10 min for medical assessment. All patients who present with a symptom complex suggestive of an acute coronary syndrome should have a 12-lead ECG completed and interpreted within a target time of 10 min of arrival at an emergency department. This allows timely decisions to be made with regard to thrombolysis and revascularization procedures. However, such triage is still dependent on non-specialist application of diagnostic tests.

LIMITATIONS OF DIAGNOSTIC TESTS

The ECG

The most important factor in the diagnosis of acute myocardial infarction is the 12-lead ECG.[16–18] The normal myocardium depolarizes from endocardium to epicardium. With the onset of coronary artery occlusion and the resultant ischaemia, changes in the pattern of depolarization occur. With acute myocardial ischaemia, a reversal of the normal direction of depolarization occurs whereby the myocardium depolarizes in the reverse order, from the normal epicardium to the endocardium. This is usually reflected by changes in the ST-segment of the ECG.

However, there are serious limitations of the ECG in the early assessment of acute chest pain. The sensitivity of a single ECG remains in the range 40–50%. The Multicentre Chest Pain Study evaluated the sensitivity of the ECG in diagnosing AMI in patients who presented to the emergency department with chest pain. Only 45% of AMI patients showed the expected ECG changes, and a further 34% showed changes consistent with ischaemia.[18]

The National Heart Attack Program (NHAP) listed the following reasons for the limitations of the standard ECG:

- If the patient has myocardial ischaemia and 'is pain free at the time when the ECG is obtained, a normal ECG may be obtained'.
- The ECG has limited ability to detect damage in the right ventricle.
- The ECG may not detect small areas of ischaemia or infarction.
- Myocardial infarction in the distribution of the circumflex artery is more likely to have non-diagnostic ECGs.[19]

The ECG has too low a sensitivity and specificity to be used as a single diagnostic test for AMI, and the value of the ECG is also operator dependent. Therefore it has serious limitations in the early assessment of potential AMI.

Serial ECGs have been advocated as having superior diagnostic performance to a single ECG. However, there are still serious diagnostic limitations with these ECGs. The same problems pertain as for the single ECG. Singer *et al.*[20] evaluated 94 patients who had an AMI with non-diagnostic ECGs. The gold standard used was the WHO criteria for diagnosis of AMI. In total, 80% showed no diagnostic change, and AMI was diagnosed on the basis of enzymes alone. If serial ECGs were utilized as an extended triage tool for the emergency department patients, then 16 out of every 100 AMI patients would be discharged inappropriately.[20]

Continuous ST-segment monitoring has also been considered in the early evaluation of these patients. It facilitates the early detection of AMI, and it will allow detection of those patients who have ST-segment instability secondary to myocardial ischaemia. Given the limitations of electrocardiography discussed previously, continuous ST-segment monitoring has too low a sensitivity (68%) to be utilized safely in isolation as a tool for ruling out myocardial infarction. However, it is a very useful clinical tool for detecting ST-segment instability.

Macromolecular markers of myocardial injury

Many biochemical markers of myocardial damage have been proposed over the years. Unfortunately, there is currently no single early myocardial marker that has a sufficiently low false-negative rate to allow an early ruling out of myocardial infarction. The three classic myocardial markers, namely creatine kinase (CK), aspartate transaminase (AST) and lactate dehydrogenase (LDH), are still commonly used. The newer markers fall into two categories, namely the classical enzyme CK-MB analysed by newer methods, and the completely new cardiac markers (e.g. the troponins).

Creatine kinase

Creatine kinase (CK) is an enzyme which catalyses the reversible transfer of phosphate from creatine phosphate to adenosine diphosphate. Its concentration usually rises within 4 h of myocardial injury. However, it can be elevated due to injury to tissues other than myocardium. It is composed of two subunits, M (muscle) and B (brain). Three isoenzymes of CK exist, namely CK-BB (CK-1) (found mainly in kidney and brain), CK-MB (CK-2) and CK-MM (CK-3) (both found mainly in muscle). Other tissues that contain CK-MB include the uterus and placenta. In addition, CK-MB levels are raised in thyroid, prostate and lung cancers.

Various biochemical tests measure CK and its isoforms. These include total CK, CK-MB, CK mass and CK isoforms. CK and CK-MB levels rise 4–8 h post infarction and return to normal 2–3 days later.

Various approaches have been tested in an attempt to improve the diagnostic accuracy of CK in the context of emergency department patients.

CK slopes initially held some promise, on the basis that the characteristic rise in CK levels in AMI patients could be used to diagnose AMI. However, in a study conducted by Leung *et al.*, the CK slope was assessed as a diagnostic tool for ruling out AMI, and this had a sensitivity of 99% but a specificity of only 74%.[21] Therefore it does not perform adequately as a diagnostic tool for this purpose.

CK-MB is an isoform of CK that is found in muscle tissue. It is measured using a classical enzymatic test similar to that for CK. The isoenzymes of CK (CK-BB, CK-MB and CK-MM) have a number of isoforms. These have been suggested to increase the diagnostic sensitivity of CK-MB. There is only one isoform of CK-MB and CK-MM in myocardium (CK-MB2 and CK-MM3). Studies on CCU patients suggest that isoforms of CK-MB are more sensitive than CK and CK-MB during the early period of evolving myocardial damage.[22]

CK-mass assays utilize monoclonal antibodies to measure the protein concentration of CK-MB, rather than the catalytic activity which is measured in conventional CK-MB assays. CK-MM, CK-BB and other compounds that interfere with CK-MB assays do not interfere with the CK-mass assay, so the number of false-positive results is reduced. Furthermore, the test reaches high levels of sensitivity at an earlier point than CK-MB.[23] To achieve 100% sensitivity in the diagnosis of cardiac pathology in a population of patients presenting to an emergency department with chest pain, the cut-off point for CK mass would be a level less than 2 mcg/L. However, the specificity of the test at this level would be only 50%. This would result in the diagnosis of an excessive number of false-positive cases. Conversely, to achieve 100% specificity the CK-MB-mass cut-off point would need to be higher than 22 mcg/L. This has a sensitivity of 38.9%, resulting in an excessive number of patients who would be inappropriately discharged.[24]

The troponins

The troponin-related complex (TRC) is a muscle-specific protein that is intrinsic to the process of contraction of muscle fibres. It is found inside the sarcomere attached to actin. Of the three proteins that make up the TRC, troponin T (TnT) and troponin I (TnI) have isoforms specific to myocardial tissue. Although the half-life of TnT is only 2 h, it can be detected in the blood for up to 2 weeks post injury. This suggests that there is a continuous release of the protein from the necrotic tissue. Studies on CCU and AMI patients have suggested that the sensitivity of TnT 10 h post pain is 100%.[22,23] TnT is an effective risk stratification tool in many groups of patients, including emergency department chest pain patients,[25] and those with unstable angina and acute myocardial ischaemia.[26] Chest pain patients with raised TnT levels are at much higher risk of AMI or death than patients with normal levels (odds ratio, 25.8; 95% CI, 9.6–48.6).

The use of early troponin T levels (two measurements in the first 6 h) to determine whether to discharge patients from the emergency department is also currently under investigation. However, most published studies have demonstrated a lack of sensitivity of early troponin T in the first 12 h after the onset of pain.[22,27]

Hamm *et al.* evaluated the clinical utility of troponin T in emergency department chest pain patients who were unsuitable for thrombolysis.[25] The paper concluded that cases with negative troponin T at 6 h after the onset of pain were a low-risk group and could be safely discharged from the emergency department. Inpatients underwent a number of investigations to rule in AMI and myocardial ischaemia. However, the discharged group was assessed by means of a telephone call to ascertain whether they had had an AMI and whether they were still alive. Therefore an independent gold standard test of myocardial damage was not applied to all cases. The methodology of follow-up for cases may have been a significant source of verification bias. Data from the Multicenter Chest Pain Study of missed AMI suggest that, using the end-point as defined in the study by Hamm *et al.*, the missed AMI rate would be 1.89% compared with 2.4% for 6-h troponin T.[22] This implies that troponin T levels in the first 6 h of pain showed no improvement over diagnosis in the late 1970s and early 1980s.

Operation of a chest pain assessment unit (CPAU)

Appropriate patient selection for admission to CPAUs will affect responses to treatment, complications and costs. CPAUs should be used for patients with a low to moderate risk of acute coronary syndrome only. The inclusion of patients who are at high risk of complications and serious comorbidity will interfere with assessment and final discharge from the CPAU.

The initial units established 10 years ago focused primarily on the safe ruling out of AMI. With the advances in technology that have taken place over the past 10 years, adjuncts such as continuous ST-segment monitoring have allowed these units to develop further and to shift their focus on early identification of AMI (ruling in myocardial infarction), as well as facilitating safe discharge of patients and a more appropriate usage of inpatient hospital resources.

This approach can also be expanded to evaluation beyond identification of myocardial necrosis, to include resting and exercise-induced myocardial ischaemia. This will enable the appropriate risk modification to be offered to patients who are now known to have a significant additional mortality from ischaemic heart disease.

THE ROLE OF EXERCISE TESTING IN CHEST PAIN ASSESSMENT UNITS

The role of exercise testing after stabilization of patients who have been admitted with unstable angina is well established. The largest reported study of exercise ECG testing as part of a chest pain assessment unit was a retrospective analysis of 1010 patients conducted by Zalenski and Grzybowski.[28] This protocol included 9 h of continuous ST-segment monitoring, serum CK-MB levels and resting ECG. Symptom-limited exercise ECG testing was performed by 78% of the patient group. The remainder of the group were not fit for discharge, as they had not successfully completed the protocol. Among this 78%, a 5% prevalence of ischaemic heart disease was identified and the 30-day mortality rate was very low. The Rapid Rule-Out of Myocardial Ischaemia Observation (ROMIO) study by Gomez *et al.*[29] prospectively evaluated 100 patients with chest pain and found very similar results. There is significant evidence that this group of patients has a longer-term additional risk of acute coronary syndromes.[30–34] Therefore it is appropriate to provide targeted secondary intervention for this group. Cardiac risk factor modification has been shown to be even more cost-effective than primary prevention in the overall fight to reduce the number of deaths from ischaemic heart disease.[3]

PATIENT SELECTION

The group of patients who are ideal for admission to CPAUs consists of those with possible cardiac chest pain, who are low-probability cases. Therefore any patient who requires direct admission to a CCU (e.g. with high-risk chest pain) should be excluded. Markers of high risk can be determined using the Goldman intensive-care filter for patients with chest pain.[16] Patients under 25 years of age are usually excluded, as the prevalence of cardiac disease below this age is very low. Chest pain that persists for longer than 12 h can be excluded, as myocardial damage can be adequately ruled out with conventional and new markers. Patient selection can be summarized as follows:

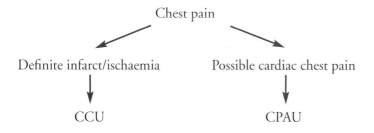

Therefore patients are to be included in the CPAU if they fulfil the following inclusion criteria:

- age > 25 years;
- no history of recent trauma;
- no other obvious cause of pain;
- chest pain of duration < 12 h.

Cases are then excluded if the following criteria are met:

- The ECG shows changes consistent with AMI.
- The ECG shows changes consistent with acute myocardial ischaemia.
- The ECG shows an acute arrhythmia.
- The patient is hypotensive.
- The patient gives a history consistent with unstable angina (defined as a patient with worsening of previous stable angina or first episode of pain post AMI or revascularization technique).
- The patient requires admission for another medical or social reason.

Summary

The evaluation of acute chest pain in the emergency department continues to pose a significant challenge to emergency physicians. The standard approach involves history taking, clinical examination, 12-lead ECG and cardiac markers, all of which have their own diagnostic limitations.[35] The assessment and management of patients who present with 'chest pain of query cardiac origin' can be enhanced through the establishment of chest pain assessment systems.

References

1. World Health Organization; www.who.int/whr/2000
2. Norris R, on behalf of the United Kingdom Heart Attack Study Collaborative Group. Fatality outside hospital from acute coronary events in three British health districts. *Br Med J* 1998; **316**: 1065–70.
3. Goldman L, Coxson P, Hunink MG *et al.* The relative influence of secondary versus primary prevention using the National Cholesterol Education Program Adult Treatment Panel II guidelines. *J Am Coll Cardiol* 1999; **34**: 768–76.
4. Fothergill NJ, Hunt MT, Touquet R. Audit of patients with chest pain presenting to an accident and emergency department over a 6-month period. *Arch Emerg Med* 1993; **10**: 155–60.

5. Emerson PA, Russell NJ, Wyatt J *et al.* An audit of doctors' management of patients with chest pain in the accident and emergency department. *Q J Med* 1989; **70**: 213–20.

6. Lee TH, Cook EF, Weisberg MC, Rouan GW, Brand DA, Goldman L. Impact of the availability of a prior electrocardiogram on the triage of the patient with acute chest pain. *J Gen Intern Med* 1990; **5**: 381–8.

7. Pope JH, Aufderheide MD, Ruthazer R *et al.* Missed diagnosis of acute myocardial ischemia in the emergency department. *N Engl J Med* 2000; **342**(16): 1163–70.

8. Killip T. Treatment of acute myocardial infarction in the coronary care unit. *Am J Cardiol* 1967; **20**: 457.

9. Bloom BS, Peterson OL. Coronary-care units. *N Engl J Med* 1973; **288**: 525–9.

10. Goldman L. Coronary care units. A perspective on their epidemiologic impact. *Int J Cardiol* 1982; **2**: 284–7.

11. Schroeder J, Lamb IH, Harrison DC. Patients admitted to the coronary care units for chest pain: a high-risk group for subsequent cardiac death. *Am J Cardiol* 1977; **39**: 829–32.

12. Wyatt J, Weber JE. A transatlantic comparison of training in emergency medicine. *J Accid Emerg Med* 1998; **15**: 363.

13. Rusnak RA, Stair TO, Hansen K, Fastow JS. Litigation against the emergency physician: common features in cases of missed myocardial infarction. *Ann Emerg Med* 1989; **18**: 1029–34.

14. Karcz A, Holbrook J, Burke MC *et al.* Massachusetts Emergency Medicine closed malpractice claims. *Ann Emerg Med* 1993; **22**: 553–9.

15. Kannel WB, Abbot RD. Incidence and prognosis of unrecognized myocardial infarction. *N Engl J Med* 1984; **311**: 1144–7.

16. Goldman L, Cook EF, Johnson PA, Brand DA, Rouan GW, Lee TH. Prediction of the need for intensive care in patients who come to the emergency departments with acute chest pain. *N Engl J Med* 1996; **334**: 1498–504.

17. Goldman L, Cook EF, Brand DA *et al.* A computer protocol to predict myocardial infarction in emergency department patients with chest pain. *N Engl J Med* 1988; **318**: 797–803.

18. Lee TH, Weisberg MC, Brand DA *et al. for* the Chest Pain Study Group. Sensitivity of routine clinical criteria for diagnosing myocardial infarction within 24 hours of hospitalization. *Ann Intern Med* 1987; **106**: 181–6.

19. Paul SD, O'Gara PT, Mahjoub ZA *et al.* Geriatric patients with acute myocardial infarction: cardiac risk profile, presentation, thrombolysis, coronary interventions and prognosis. *Am Heart J* 1996; **131**: 710–15.

20. Singer AJ, Brogan GX, Valentine SM, McCuskey C, Khan S, Hollander JE. Effect of duration from symptom onset on the negative

predictive value of a normal ECG for exclusion of acute myocardial infarction. *Ann Emerg Med* 1997; **29**: 575–9.

21. Leung FY, Griffith AP, Jablonsky G, Henderson AR. Comparison of the diagnostic utility of timed serial (slope) creatine kinase measurements with conventional serum tests in the early diagnosis of myocardial infarction. *Ann Clin Biochem* 1991; **28**: 78–82.

22. Mair J, Morandell D, Genser N, Lechleitner P, Dienstl F, Puschendorf B. Equivalent early sensitivities of myoglobin, creatine kinase MB mass, creatine kinase isoform ratios and cardiac troponins I and T for acute myocardial infarction. *Clin Chem* 1995; **41**: 1266–72.

23. Mair J. Progress in myocardial damage detection: new biochemical markers for clinicians. *Crit Rev Lab Sci* 1997; **34**: 1–66.

24. Herren R, Mackway-Jones K, Richards R, Senerviratne CJ, France MW, Cotter L. Diagnostic cohort study of an emergency department-based 6-hour rule-out protocol for myocardial damage. *Br Med J* 2001; **323**: 1–4.

25. Hamm CW, Goldmann BU, Heeschen G, Berger J, Meinertz T. Emergency-room triage of patients with acute chest pain by means of rapid testing for cardiac troponin T or troponin I. *N Engl J Med* 1997; **337**: 1648–53.

26. Christenson RH, Duh SH, Newby LK *et al.* Cardiac troponin T and cardiac troponin I: relative values in short-term risk stratification of patients with acute coronary syndromes. *Clin Chem* 1998; **44**: 494–501.

27. Bakker AJ, Koelemay MJW, Gorgels JPMC *et al.* Failure of biochemical markers to exclude acute myocardial infarction at admission. *Lancet* 1993; **342**: 1220–2.

28. Zalenski RJ, Grzybowski M. The chest pain centre in the emergency department. *Emerg Med Clin North Am* 2001; **19**: 469–81.

29. Gomez MA, Anderson JL, Karagounis LS *et al.* An emergency department-based protocol for rapidly ruling out myocardial ischemia reduces hospital waiting times: ROMIO study. *J Am Coll Cardiol* 1996; **28**: 25–33.

30. Launbjerg J. The long-term prognosis of patients with acute chest pain, but without myocardial infarction. *Dan Med Bull* 1997; **44**: 365–79.

31. Launbjerg J, Fruergaard P, Hesse B, Jorgensen F, Elsborg L, Petri A. Long-term risk of death, cardiac events and recurrent chest pain in patients with acute chest pain of different origin. *Cardiology* 1996; **87**: 60–6.

32. Launbjerg J, Fruergaard P, Madsen JK, Mortensen LS, Hansen JF. Ten-year mortality of patients admitted to coronary care units with and without myocardial infarction. Risk factors from medical history

and diagnosis at discharge. Danish Verapamil Infarction Trial. *Cardiology* 1994; **85**: 259–66.

33. Lee TH, Ting HH, Shammash JB, Soukup JR, Goldman L. Long-term survival of emergency department patients with acute chest pain. *Am J Cardiol* 1992; **69**: 145–51.

34. Goldman L. Using prediction models and cost-effectiveness analysis to improve clinical decisions: emergency department patients with acute chest pain. *Proc Assoc Am Physicians* 1995; **107**: 329–33.

35. Balk EM, Ioannidis JPA, Salem D *et al.* Accuracy of biomarkers to diagnose acute cardiac ischemia in the emergency department: a meta-analysis. *Ann Emerg Med* 2001; **37**: 478–94.

Investigations

Ross T. Murphy

Introduction

Many clinicians are faced with the unenviable task of diagnosing angina without any specific training in the battery of complex and expensive tests now available. These investigations have been modified and refined during the last decade, and a reasonably widely held consensus is emerging as to which investigations to use and in what order. In this chapter we have tried to organize these investigations into an acceptable order of priority. We have also emphasized the sensitivity and specificity of each modality in particular situations. While national and international guidelines have their place, the clinician must also take into account local experience and expertise, cost, and the frequency with which certain tests are performed. One must always stress the importance of clinical history and examination, without which no investigation has any meaning.

Electrocardiogram

A resting electrocardiogram (ECG) is a simple initial investigation. Although this is of low sensitivity in determining underlying coronary disease, an abnormal resting ECG at presentation does identify a group of patients with coronary heart disease with a poorer long-term outcome. However, it is normal in well over 50% of patients who have symptoms consistent with angina pectoris. A normal resting ECG (see Figure 8.1) does not preclude severe coronary disease. Evidence of Q-waves makes the diagnosis of ischaemic heart disease (IHD) quite likely. The ECG may also identify patients with atrial fibrillation and ventricular dysrhythmia.

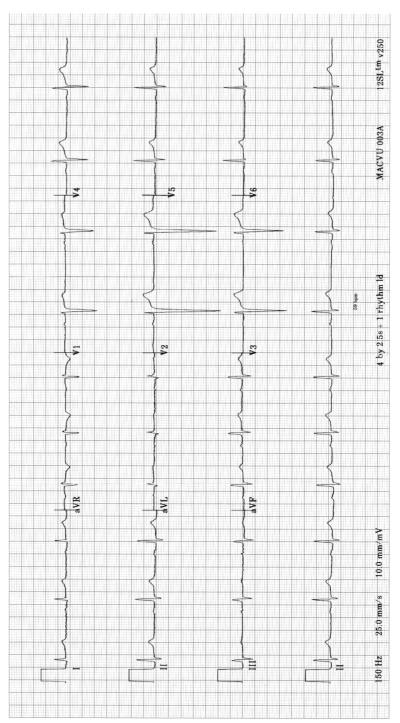

Figure 8.1
Normal ECG at rest.

On the other hand, an ECG obtained during pain is quite useful (see Figure 8.2), and is abnormal in over 50% of patients with angina who have a normal resting ECG. Many high-risk patients with ECG changes during pain require no further non-invasive investigations.

Exercise testing

The exercise stress test (EST) is the most important non-invasive investigation for patients with angina pectoris. It can provide objective evidence of the presence of disease, and is an independent predictor of cardiovascular death. It is cheap and has been in widespread clinical use for several decades. Several standard protocols are now widely used (see Table 8.1), and both treadmill and bicycle ergometers are acceptable methods of assessing exercise capacity. Treadmills are used more commonly, as bicycle ergometers often cause fatigue of the quadriceps muscles before maximum exercise capacity is reached. Ideally, the protocol should be chosen to permit the patient to exercise for between 6 and 12 min, and should express exercise capacity in metabolic equivalents (MET) (where 1 MET refers to VO_2 at a standard basal uptake rate of 3.5 L/kg per min).

Exercise testing should include monitoring of the heart rate and blood pressure during each stage of the standard protocol and during ST change and/or chest pain. There should be ongoing monitoring for ST-segment change and transient arrhythmias. Recent American Heart Association/American College of Cardiology (AHA/ACC) guidelines suggest that all exercise testing should be supervised by an appropriately trained physician.[1] The incidence of death and/or myocardial infarction during and just after exercise testing has been reported to be as high as 1 in 2500 tests.[2]

Absolute contraindications to exercise testing include the following:

- myocardial infarction within 2 days;
- severe aortic stenosis;
- symptomatic severe heart failure;
- pericarditis;
- symptomatic arrhythmias or those causing haemodynamic compromise.

Relative contraindications include the following:

- moderate aortic stenosis;
- systolic blood pressure > 200 mmHg, or diastolic pressure > 110 mmHg;
- hypertrophic cardiomyopathy with severe outflow obstruction.

Exercise testing may be terminated when one of a number of endpoints is reached.

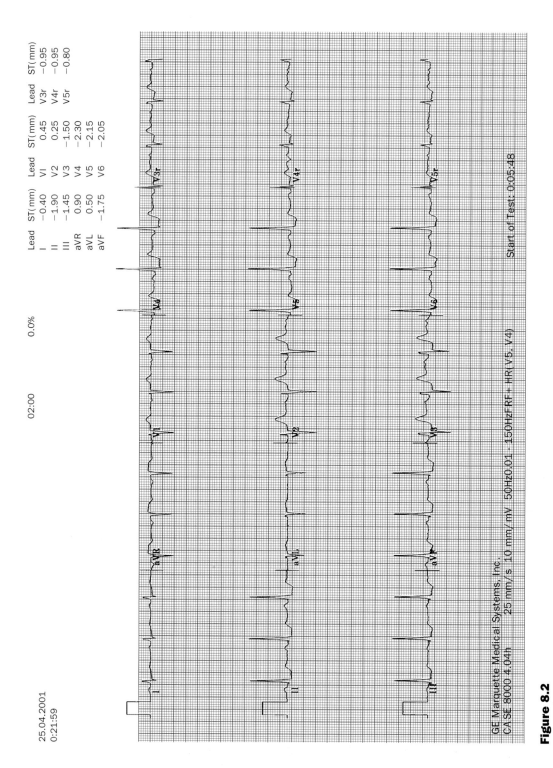

25.04.2001
0:21:59

02:00

0.0%

Lead	ST (mm)	Lead	ST (mm)	Lead	ST (mm)
I	−0.40	V1	0.45	V3r	−0.95
II	−1.90	V2	0.25	V4r	−0.95
III	−1.45	V3	−1.50	V5r	−0.80
aVR	0.90	V4	−2.30		
aVL	0.50	V5	−2.15		
aVF	−1.75	V6	−2.05		

GE Marquette Medical Systems, Inc.
CASE 8000 4.04h   25 mm/s 10 mm/mV 50Hz0.01 -150HzFRF+ HR(V5, V4)   Start of Test 0:05:48

Figure 8.2
ECG during angina pectoris with significant widespread ST depression.

Protocol	Starts	Finishes
Bruce (stages at 3-min intervals)	1.7 mph at 10% gradient (5 MET)	5.5 mph at 20% gradient (16 MET)
Modified Bruce (two introductory stages)	1.7 mph at 0% gradient (5 MET)	5.5 mph at 20% gradient (16 MET)
Naughton (stages at 2-min intervals)	2 mph at 0% gradient (2 MET)	3.4 mph at 26% gradient (16 MET)

Table 8.1
Exercise protocols

Reasons for stopping EST can be summarized as follows:

- a drop in systolic blood pressure of >10 mmHg from baseline;
- moderate to severe angina;
- 2 mm downsloping or horizontal ST-segment depression;
- sustained ventricular tachycardia;
- a rise in ST segment of >1 mm in the absence of pathological Q-waves in those leads;
- systolic blood pressure >250 mmHg, or diastolic blood pressure >115 mmHg;
- fatigue, leg cramps and patient distress.

The Borg scale of perceived physical exertion[3] may be used to standardize patient responses to exercise testing. This uses a patient-directed score ranging from 6 to 7 (extremely light) to 19 to 20 (extremely hard).

The most useful changes of a positive exercise test may be taken as ≥ 1 mm horizontal or downsloping ST-segment depression 60 to 80 ms after the end of the QRS complex, during or after exercise (see Figure 8.3). Other important changes include the occurrence of chest pain consistent with angina, a drop in systolic blood pressure, ST-segment elevation in the absence of Q-waves, or sustained ventricular arrhythmias. It is important to note that the patient with well-established severe coronary disease may well have little or no ECG changes, due to well-developed collaterals or ischaemic preconditioning.

One of the most robust prognostic markers during an exercise test is maximum exercise capacity. This is measured by maximum workload achieved, maximum MET level achieved, maximum exercise duration or maximum heart rate and blood pressure product. The particular variable is unimportant. However, the inclusion of some measure of exercise capacity in the final assessment does provide a standard tool with which to risk-stratify a particular patient. ST-segment depression or elevation during exercise, as well as exercise-induced hypotension, also provides useful prognostic information. These data are best summarized using the Duke treadmill score, which is calculated as the

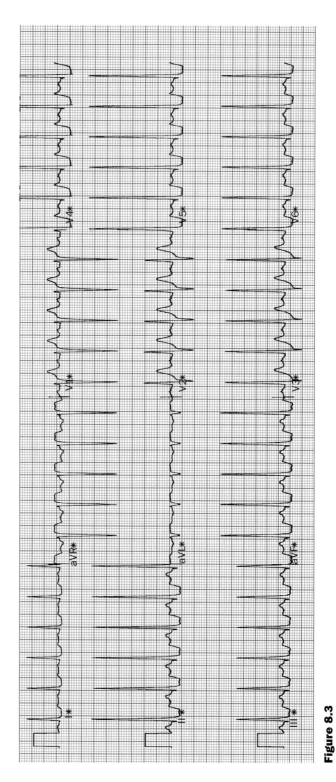

Figure 8.3
ECG at maximal stress with inferolateral ST change suggestive of reversible ischaemia in a dominant right coronary artery.

exercise time in minutes minus five times the ST-segment deviation in milli-metres minus four times the angina index, where 0 = no angina, 1 = angina, and 2 = angina being the reason for stopping the test. This simple and clin-ically relevant technique can be used to estimate average annual cardiac mortality.[4] A Duke score of less than −10 is associated with an annual mor-tality of 5%, whereas a score of ≥5 carries an annual mortality of 0.25%. Patients with a calculated mortality risk of >3% should be referred for cardiac catherization, on prognostic grounds alone.

$$
\begin{aligned}
\textit{Duke treadmill score} = {} & \text{exercise time (min)} \\
& - (5 \times \text{ST-segment deviation (mm)}) \\
& - (4 \times \text{angina index}).
\end{aligned}
$$

Estimates of the specificity and sensitivity of exercise testing have varied widely, even allowing for differences in technique and local expertise. Such *post-hoc* assessments of specificity and sensitivity are fraught with the prob-lems of assessing a test solely on the grounds of subsequent referral for a more accurate test – in this case, the gold standard of coronary angiography. This post-test referral bias can also occur when patients with a positive test are referred for angiography and those with a negative test are not. This raises the apparent sensitivity but lowers the apparent specificity of the test. The mean sensitivity for coronary disease was 68% and the mean specificity was 77% in one published meta-analysis of 24 074 exercise tests, but the range was very wide.[5] When the analysis was restricted to patients who were to have both exercise testing and angiography, the sensitivity of exercise testing for IHD was only 50%, but the specificity was 90%. False-positive tests are more com-mon in women. Exercise testing is at its most useful when the clinical risk of coronary disease is of intermediate probability, but there is little agreement about what constitutes the boundaries of intermediate probability. Clearly, clinical judgement by the individual physician is still of paramount impor-tance when analysing the exercise test.

Several specific factors affect the analysis of exercise-induced ST-segment change.

- Digoxin produces abnormal exercise ST changes in 25–40% of appar-ently normal subjects.
- Beta-blockers may mask ischaemic ST change, and should be stopped at least five half-lives before a diagnostic test, and ideally withdrawn gradu-ally to avoid rebound ischaemia.
- Pre-existing left bundle branch block (LBBB) is often associated with ST depression during exercise, without underlying ischaemia.
- Right bundle branch block (RBBB) can lead to similarly benign ST change in leads V_1 to V_3 during exercise, but ST change in the lateral or inferior leads in this context does represent potential ischaemia.

- Left ventricular hypertrophy with strain pattern is also associated with more false-positive results.
- ST-segment change during exercise has been found to be less specific and less sensitive in women. Putative reasons for this include the higher incidence of mitral valve prolapse in women, differences in microvascular function, syndrome X and the effects of oestrogen on endothelial function. Syndrome X in this context refers to women with typical angina pain, typical ECG changes on exercise stress testing, and a normal coronary angiogram. The prognosis is excellent, and although there is controversy as to whether these changes represent microvascular ischaemia or endothelial dysfunction, the response to anti-anginals is often poor. Although some clinicians favour stress imaging techniques when assessing female patients, insufficient data are available to allow one approach to be favoured over the other.

Although exercise testing is frequently limited by the patient's physical frailty, and despite its limited sensitivity, it remains the investigation of choice for the patient with suspected coronary disease. It is cheap, widely available and standardized, and is of important diagnostic and prognostic utility.

Myocardial perfusion scanning

This very different mode of investigation for coronary disease relies not on ST change but on imaging the myocardium at peak exercise and at rest. Typically this involves injection at peak exercise (or during peak stress induced chemically by dipyridamole or adenosine) of a radionuclide which is then taken up by the myocardium. The image created depends on the distribution of the radionuclide by regional blood flow. Usually this is a two-part process with a first image produced at peak stress and a second one produced at rest. If the regional blood flow is limited by a fixed stenosis, a defect on imaging will improve at rest (reversible defect). If the defect is similar at rest and at peak stress/exercise (fixed defect), this may represent an infarcted area.

From these principles was developed the discipline of myocardial perfusion scanning, which represents an important, albeit more expensive, alternative to exercise testing. It is utilized in cases where exercise testing is ruled out by physical incapacity or an abnormal resting ECG, or where the exercise test is equivocal and angiography is not immediately indicated. The costs of equipment and highly trained personnel, concerns about patient exposure to radiation, and a lack of co-ordination in developing services in some countries have meant that perfusion scanning remains an under-utilized alternative to conventional exercise testing.

Myocardial perfusion imaging uses either planar or, more recently, single photon emission computed tomography (SPECT) (see Plate 8.1) images. The injected radionuclides most commonly utilized are thallium and technetium. The peak stressor can be either exercise or the pharmacological stress of intravenous adenosine or dipyridamole, which act as coronary vasodilators. Both cause a marked increase in coronary flow, and both are associated with frequent mild side-effects, such as nausea, headache, angina, flushing, dizziness and shortness of breath. However, serious effects are rare (< 2%). The latter include arrhythmias and bronchospasm, which can be reversed by theophyllines.

Radionuclides for perfusion scanning include the following:

- thallium ^{201}TI sestamibi – redistribution allows single-injection study;
- technetium ^{99m}Tc tetrofosmin – two injections are required, but this radionuclide allows assessment of pump function;
- technetium ^{99m}Tc sestamibi.

Myocardial perfusion imaging has a relatively high sensitivity (80%) and specificity (92%) for coronary disease, and remains consistently more sensitive than exercise testing. Quantitative rather than visual analysis has been reported to increase sensitivity further, and SPECT scanning results in a sensitivity approaching 90%. A normal perfusion study carries an excellent prognosis, with a 1-year cardiac event rate of < 1%.

Several factors interfere with the diagnostic accuracy of perfusion imaging.

- Beta-blockers limit the sensitivity of the test and, as for exercise testing, beta-blockers should be withheld where possible for five half-lives before the perfusion scan.
- Occasional reports suggest that LBBB is associated with perfusion defects in the interventricular septum in the absence of coronary disease. The reasons for this are unclear, and the results of published reports are conflicting.
- Breast attenuation, especially in obese women using thallium as the radionuclide, can produce artefacts. This seems to be less of a problem with technetium and SPECT scanning.
- Very obese patients remain a problem, as most imaging tables have limits (usually *c.* 135 kg or 22 stone).

Positron emission tomography (PET)

This relatively new modality provides images of coronary blood flow and cardiac metabolism (see Plate 8.2). It uses positron-emitting radionuclides and detects paired photons emitted on collision with an electron ('annihilation'). It gives intrinsically clearer pictures than previous techniques, allows for correction of attenuation (a major advance on previous techniques) and gives a much lower radiation dose to the patient. The most widely used isotope is ^{18}F-labelled fluorodeoxyglucose (FDG), which is utilized to measure glucose metabolism in tissues. The device requires an expensive detector and access to a cyclotron to produce the isotope. These techniques are unique in that they allow quantitation of tracer concentration and therefore accurate and reproducible measures of coronary blood flow. PET may aid in excluding ischaemia in patients with chest pain and angiographically normal arteries, suggesting micovascular dysfunction.[6,7] It has been shown to be comparable, if not superior, to SPECT scanning in the detection of coronary disease, but cost remains a major obstacle to its widespread clinical utilization.

Stress echocardiography

Stress echocardiography is a sensitive and specific tool for detecting reversible ischaemia in patients with coronary stenoses. It involves imaging by two-dimensional echocardiography of localized areas of myocardium under pharmacological stress. The left ventricle is divided into 16 segments, and wall motion is scored according to an arbitrary system where 1 = normal motion and wall thickening, 2 = hypokinetic (reduced motion and thickening), 3 = akinetic and 4 = dyskinetic (outward systolic motion and thinning). Features suggestive of ischaemia include the following:

- a decrease in normal thickening of left ventricular (LV) wall with pharmacological stress;
- a decrease in more than one segment of LV wall motion with pharmacological stress;
- areas of hyperkinesis in adjacent LV wall segments during stress.

Several agents are in common usage as pharmacological stressors. Dobutamine stress echo has significantly higher accuracy than adenosine or dipyridamole echo, and can produce substantial wall motion changes. Dobutamine increases heart rate, systolic blood pressure and myocardial contractility at higher doses, increasing coronary blood flow to two-fold or three-fold higher than baseline values. Side-effects include dizziness, headache, paraesthesiae, tremor and anxiety, but serious adverse events are rare. Dipyridamole blocks re-uptake of endogenous adenosine, thus allowing accumulation of adenosine with vascular smooth-muscle relaxation and vasodilatation. This causes a slight fall in blood pressure and a reflex rise in heart rate. Adenosine is a potent vasodilator and increases coronary blood flow.

A recent meta-analysis of a number of studies suggests a sensitivity and specificity for the detection of coronary disease of 82% and 85%, respectively.[8] The development of simultaneous four-screen storage and looped playback facilitates more accurate assessment of LV wall changes. Clearly, local expertise and experience play an important role in defining the accuracy of wall motion and thickness. There are fewer published data on the long-term prognostic value of a negative dobutamine stress echo compared with perfusion scanning or exercise testing.

Electron beam computed tomography (EBCT)

Conventional CT has a well-established role in the diagnosis of structural changes in the heart, particularly in the pericardium, and in the assessment of tumours. Normal cardiac and respiratory motion was a major obstacle to the assessment of smaller structures such as the coronary arteries, but these problems have been largely overcome in the last decade by the utilization of techniques such as EBCT, which allows rapid image acquisition without moving the source in an arc around the patient. This is achieved by an electron beam that is deflected to generate a fan of X-rays around the target. Coronary calcification is normally associated with atheroma, and it has become possible to score the density and extent of calcium deposits in a semi-quantitative manner. Although it is not of great utility in defining high-grade stenoses, EBCT has very rapidly gained a place in the screening of asymptomatic individuals who are at high risk for coronary disease, particularly in the USA. Some studies have shown that high calcium scores are associated with an increased risk of developing overt coronary heart disease, and recent research demonstrated that statin therapy may lead to a slowing of the rate of progression.[9] Although EBCT is attractive because of its non-invasive nature, at the time of writing it remains a screening tool rather than an accurate diagnostic modality.

Magnetic resonance angiography (MRA)

MRA shows great potential as a diagnostic tool for coronary artery disease and for high-grade stenoses, with huge advances in image quality having been achieved in the last few years. Images are obtained by applying a powerful magnetic field that temporarily realigns the magnetic field of protons within the subject. The restoration of normal polarity by the subject's protons is associated with a radio-signal which can then be read and processed as an image. The images produced represent the most exciting advance in cardiovascular imaging in the last decade (see Figure 8.4). High-resolution

Figure 8.4
Magnetic resonance angiogram showing coronary arteries enhanced by peripheral intravenous contrast.

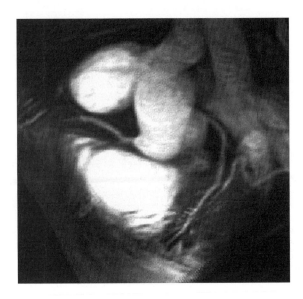

pictures of the coronary vasculature have been achieved in the last 3 years, with sensitivities of up to 88%, particularly for proximal large-vessel stenoses. However, there are still major difficulties in correcting for motion artefact, cardiac and respiratory motion.

Rapid improvements in stress magnetic resonance imaging (MRI) (using gadolinium) and in the detection of areas of myocardial infarction will ensure an important place for MRI/MRA in the very near future, although the cost and availability of MR units will be a major factor in limiting the use of this technique in the health-care systems of Western Europe.

Coronary angiography

Invasive coronary angiography remains the gold standard for detecting and assessing coronary heart disease (see Figure 8.7). First performed by Sones in 1959, it is the most commonly utilized modality for defining coronary disease. Over one million coronary angiograms are performed each year in the USA, and although angiography was initially merely a diagnostic tool, it has reinvented itself as percutaneous coronary intervention, angioplasty and stenting have been developed during the last two decades.

The procedure is discussed more fully in Chapter 9 (p. 131) and Chapter 10 (p. 153); it is still the mainstay of accurate and definitive diagnosis of significant coronary artery obstruction. Important advances have changed our understanding of atherosclerosis from the concept of a passive accumulation of lipids with flow-limiting stenoses to one of global endothelial dysfunction,

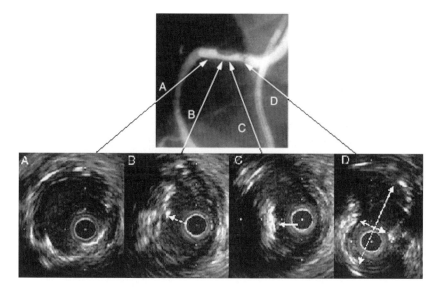

Figure 8.5
Intravascular ultrasound (IVUS) scan revealing significant plaque burden in an angiographically patent vessel.

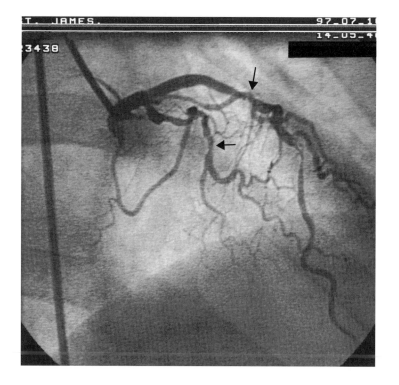

Figure 8.6
Coronary angiogram: left anterior descending and circumflex artery with severe disease in both vessels.

with plaque stability being a major factor in clinical presentation. Glagov[10] showed that early atherosclerosis tends to cause a compensatory vessel remodelling outwards, which preserves luminal size and is undetectable at angiography. The use of intravascular ultrasound (IVUS) probes has revealed

Figure 8.7
Coronary angiogram: right coronary artery with severe disease, pre- and post angioplasty and stenting.

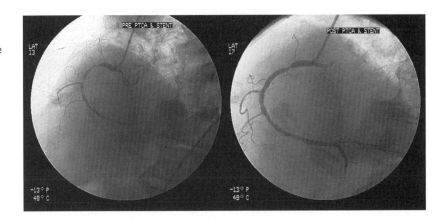

that much of the atherosclerotic burden of a coronary artery remains undetected by conventional angiography, and that the 'luminogram' that arteriography produces does not give an accurate picture of the total plaque burden or of the true biological state of a vessel (see Figure 8.5). Elective coronary angiography is usually performed as a day case procedure and the use of brachial and radial artery access has facilitated early mobilization compared with the traditional femoral artery approach. Accurate visualization of the extent and severity of coronary atheroma allows planning of angioplasty or surgery. Complication rates from elective coronary angiography are low, with a mortality/peri-procedural myocardial infarction/stroke rate of <1%, and access site complications, including pseudoaneurysm formation of 1–2%. Nonetheless, coronary angiography is well established and widely available, and it remains the gold standard for diagnosis and assessment of coronary artery disease (see Figures 8.6 and 8.7).

References

1. American College of Cardiology/American Heart Association/American College of Physicians/Association of Internal Medicine. Guidelines for the management of chronic stable angina. *J Am Coll Cardiol* 1999; **33**: 2093–197.
2. Stuart RJ, Ellestad MH. National survey of exercise testing facilities. *Chest* 1980; **77**: 94–7.
3. Borg GA. Psychophysical bases of perceived exertion. *Med Sci Sports Exerc* 1982; **14**: 377–82.
4. Mark DB, Shaw L, Harrel FE *et al.* Prognostic value of a treadmill exercise score in outpatients with suspected coronary artery disease. *N Engl J Med* 1991; **325**: 849–53.
5. Gibbons RJ, Balady GJ, Beasley JW *et al.* ACC/AHA guidelines for exercise training. Executive summary. *Circulation* 1997; **96**: 345–54.

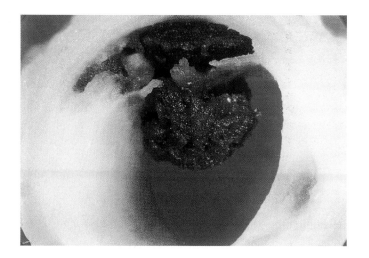

Plate 3.1
Plaque rupture: cross-section of a coronary plaque with rupture of plaque wall and spread of thrombus occluding the main lumen, resulting in a fatal myocardial infarction. Reproduced with permission from the American Heart Association. Davies MJ. *Circulation* 1995; **95**: 2846.

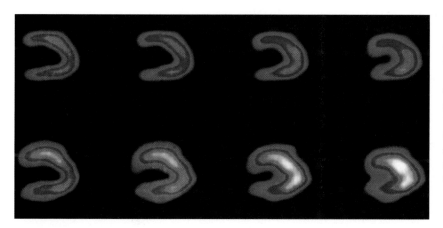

Plate 8.1
Radionuclide stress test (TC-MIBI) showing decreased uptake in upper row (exercise) compared with lower row (rest), suggesting reversible ischaemia in the anterior surface (vertical long axis) supplied by left anterior descending artery. Courtesy Dr G. Duffy.

SHORT AXIS

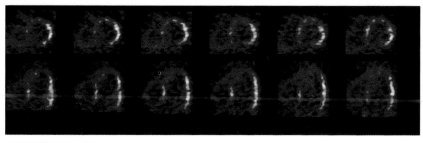

HORIZONTAL LONG AXIS

Plate 8.2
^{18}FDG-gated positron emission tomogram (PET) allowing accurate quantification of glucose metabolism and blood flow with a lower radiation dose, here showing decreased uptake in the apex and septum, indicating an old infarct.

Plate 10.1
Concentric narrowing of a
coronary artery lumen by a
large lipid-laden plaque.
Reproduced with
permission of
BMJ Publishing Group.
Davies MJ. *Heart* 2000;
83(2): 363.

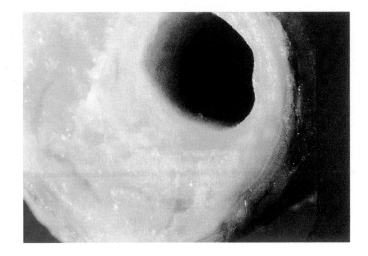

6. Camici PG, Gropler RJ, Jones T *et al*. The impact of myocardial blood flow quantitation with PET on the understanding of cardiac disease. *Eur Heart J* 1996; **17**: 25–34.

7. Camici PG. PET and myocardial imaging. *Heart* 2000; **83**: 475–80.

8. Cheitlin MD, Alpert JS, Armstrong *et al*. ACC/AHA guidelines for the clinical application of echocardiography. *Circulation* 1997: **96**: 345–54.

9. Callister TO, Raggi P, Cooil P *et al*. Effect of HMGCoA reductase inhibitors on coronary artery disease as assessed by EBCT. *N Engl J Med* 1998; **339**: 1972–8.

10. Glagov S. Hemodynamic risk factors, mechanical stress, mural architecture, medial nutrition and the vulnerability of arteries to atherosclerosis. In: *The pathogenesis of atherosclerosis*. Baltimore, MD: Williams and Wilkins, 1972: 164–89.

Management of chronic stable angina

Robert Kelly and Peter Crean

Introduction

Chronic stable angina is defined as retrosternal chest discomfort due to myocardial ischaemia. Characteristically it is precipitated by physical exertion and/or emotional stress. It is often described as a pressure or strangling sensation, lasting for 1–15 min and usually relieved rapidly by rest or taking nitrates. It may radiate to the neck, shoulders, jaw, back or arms (usually the left arm). Angina is said to be stable if it occurs over a period of several weeks without deteriorating. Cold weather, heavy meals, tachycardia or fever may exacerbate the symptoms. The presence of risk factors such as smoking, diabetes mellitus or hypertension makes the diagnosis of angina more likely (see Box 9.1). During angina episodes, patients may appear pale and sweaty, with a tachycardia and an apical systolic murmur due to mitral regurgitation, or a third heart sound. It is important when examining these patients to identify signs of risk factors, such as xanthomata, as well as ruling out other potential causes of angina symptoms, such as aortic stenosis, anaemia and hypertension.

In a subgroup of patients, angina may occur with normal coronary anatomy. This is called syndrome X, and is usually observed in obese female patients with metabolic abnormalities. There are observations which suggest that these patients may have endothelial dysfunction. The prognosis with regard to mortality is generally good, but these patients tend to respond poorly to conventional medical therapy.

Angina pectoris is prevalent in 2–8% of the general population, with an increased prevalence being attributable to the ageing population.[1] Men are affected more than women. The incidence ranges from 0.44 per 1000 per year (age 31–40 years) to 2.3 per 1000 per year (age 60 years) in men, and from 0.8 per 1000 per year to 1.1 per 1000 per year in women.[2] In the UK, this amounts to 22 000 new cases of angina per year. The annual risk of a major cardiac

> **Box 9.1   Risk factors for coronary artery disease**
>
> - Smoking
> - Diet
> - Lack of exercise
> - Cholesterol level > 5.0 mmol/L
> - Positive family history
> - Hypertension
> - Diabetes/glucose intolerance

event (death or myocardial infarction) in chronic stable angina is 2%.[3] Around 25% of patients with a myocardial infarction (MI) have a previous history of angina, and patients with symptoms of angina are at increased risk of infarction compared with patients with asymptomatic coronary artery disease. Sudden death is also more common among patients with chronic stable angina.[4]

Aetiology

Angina results from the partial obstruction of a coronary artery by atherosclerosis. The latter is precipitated by risk factors such as hypertension, cigarette smoking, diabetes and hyperlipidaemia.[2–4] The atheroma may be present without causing any symptoms. Angina occurs due to an imbalance between myocardial oxygen supply and demand. The supply of oxygen is affected by obstruction of a coronary artery due to atheroma. Myocardial oxygen demand is determined by heart rate, contractility, left ventricular (LV) systolic pressure and volume. Changes in vasomotor tone may also induce ischaemia, causing vasoconstriction of normal coronary arteries (coronary spasm). Platelet aggregation on sites of atherosclerosis will also precipitate ischaemia.

Prognosis

The prognosis for stable angina patients is generally favourable. However, it is important to identify a number of factors so that appropriate therapy can be targeted early for certain patients. This is especially the case with high-risk patients, who are more likely to benefit from surgery or angioplasty. Angina patients at high risk may be identified on the basis of the factors listed in Box 9.2.

Box 9.2   Factors associated with an adverse prognosis

- *Age:* Older patients are at increased risk for fatal and non-fatal cardiac events.
- *Gender:* Men are at greater risk than women, although this risk is the same after menopause.
- *Symptoms:* Poor exercise tolerance due to pain (which may arise from ischaemia or left ventricular dysfunction) identifies higher-risk patients, who are likely to benefit most from revascularization. It should be remembered that patients' symptoms do not correlate well with the severity/progression of coronary artery stenoses.
- *ECG changes:* Pain and ST-segment depression double the risk for coronary events. Previous MI, especially Q-waves on an ECG, are associated with higher risk.
- *LV systolic function:* LV systolic dysfunction/ejection fraction below 40% on multiple uptake gated acquisition scan (MUGA)/echocardiography (ECHO) at rest or on exercise worsens the prognosis.
- *Exercise ECG:* ST-segment depression > 2 mm increases morbidity. ST-segment depression > 3 mm is associated with left main stem and three-vessel disease.
- *Exercise ECG:* Chronotropic incompetence with exercise and a fall in blood pressure on exercise confer an increase in risk.
- *Perfusion scan:* Thallium uptake in the lungs on perfusion scans confers an increase in risk.
- *Angiography:* Increased risk is associated with the severity and extent of coronary disease (i.e. left main stem involvement, proximal left anterior descending artery stenosis, and multi-vessel disease, especially in the presence of LV systolic dysfunction).

Medical treatment of chronic stable angina

Medical treatment of patients with chronic stable angina has two aims:

1. to improve the prognosis by preventing MI and death;
2. to minimize or relieve symptoms.

The approach includes secondary prevention, medical therapy and revascularization.[5]

SECONDARY PREVENTION

Risk factor modification is the cornerstone of management of patients with angina pectoris (see Chapter 12, page 177).

Smoking cessation

Smoking cessation is crucial for patients with angina. In the Western world, 50% of all mortality is attributable to smoking. Those patients who continue to smoke risk reducing the effectiveness of medical therapy, and will increase their complication rate from angioplasty or bypass surgery. Smoking will also increase angina symptoms.

It is now recognized that smoking is a true addiction, and better response rates to smoking cessation may be achieved by treating it as such. Encouragement is required, and useful sources of support, such as Stop Smoking Clinics and advice lines, as well as nicotine replacement therapies should be easily accessible. Newer therapies directed at treating nicotine dependency (e.g. buproprion) may help to improve smoking cessation,[6] although safety issues have recently been highlighted, together with the potential for pro-arrhythmia in some patients.

Diet

A low-fat, low-cholesterol diet with a fat intake below 30% of calorific intake is advised. In overweight patients, a weight-reducing diet is required. Weight reduction should aim for a waist circumference of <94 cm in men and <80 cm in women. Vigorous lifestyle modification has been shown to result in regression of coronary artery disease. A healthy diet can reduce cardiac mortality by 42% and all-cause mortality by 45%.[7] It is equally important to moderate alcohol intake and restrict salt intake.

Exercise

Increased exercise improves the ischaemic threshold, and 30 min of exercise four or five times per week is recommended. The exercise capacity of individual patients can be assessed by formal exercise ECG testing.

Psychological factors

Reassurance, relaxation and patient education are all very important. Patients who are not already stressed will commonly become so when their angina is diagnosed. Issues about quality of life are also important. Angina will often limit quality of life according to the patient's perception of their illness. Patients believe that the severity of comorbid illness, their anticipated relief of symptoms and how they rate angina-free treatment determine their quality of life more than any symptoms of angina. Quality of life may be improved

---

Box 9.3   Drugs with prognostic benefit in stable angina

Antiplatelets

- Aspirin, 75 mg
- Clopidogrel, 75 mg

Statins

- Atorvastatin, 10–80 mg
- Fluvastatin, 20–40 mg
- Pravastatin, 10–40 mg
- Simvastatin, 20–80 mg

---

if patients are told to avoid triggering factors such as heavy meals, cold weather and strenuous exercise. In the UK, work such as heavy goods vehicle driving or bus driving is contraindicated in patients with angina pectoris,[8] but car driving is permitted. Sexual intercourse may trigger angina, so common sense is advised. Nitrate prophylaxis may help. The use of Viagra in patients with stable angina is permitted, though not wih concomitant nitrate therapy.[9] It is important to remember that medical and surgical treatment aims to improve quality of life in angina patients.

MEDICAL THERAPY TO IMPROVE PROGNOSIS

Antiplatelet and lipid-lowering therapy improve the prognosis (see Box 9.3). Beta-blockers reduce mortality following MI. Although nitrates, calcium-channel blockers and beta-blockers give symptom relief to angina patients, there is no evidence that they prolong life or reduce mortality in individuals with chronic stable angina.[10–12]

Aspirin and clopidogrel

Mechanism of action (see Figure 9.1)

Aspirin irreversibly acetylates cyclo-oxygenase, and activity is not restored until new platelets are formed. Platelets cannot synthesize new proteins, so aspirin removes all of the platelet cyclo-oxygenase activity for the lifespan of the platelet. Aspirin also stops the production of thromboxane A_2, and in the vascular endothelium it inactivates cyclo-oxygenase, decreasing the formation of prostacyclin (see Figure 9.1). The overwhelming clinical effect of aspirin is antithrombotic.[13]

Clopidogrel is an ADP-receptor antagonist with a potent antiplatelet effect.

Figure 9.1

Mechanism of action of aspirin and clopidogrel.

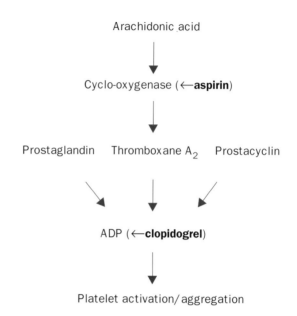

Aspirin is hydrolysed to salicylic acid, which is only a weak inactivator of cyclo-oxygenase with a half-life of 2–3 h, compared with 20 min for aspirin. Although low doses of aspirin (e.g. 20 mg) have a documented platelet-inhibitory effect, the problem with such doses is that the full antithrombotic effect takes up to 48 h to develop. In contrast, standard doses are effective within hours.

Clinical effects

In stable angina pectoris, aspirin 75 mg daily reduces the risk of acute MI and sudden death by 34% (Swedish SAPAT study).[14] In smaller studies, 325 mg of aspirin given on alternate days has been shown to reduce the risk of acute MI by 87% when taken for 5 years.[15] Similarly, in ISIS-2, 325 mg aspirin reduced morbidity and mortality by 20%.[16] This benefit of aspirin therapy was still present after 10 years of treatment. In general, a dose of aspirin in the range 75–325 mg is clinically effective. The lower dose is preferred because of the apparent dose-related side-effects, such as gastrointestinal bleeding, which are reduced by 40% when low-dose aspirin is used.

For patients who are truly unable to tolerate aspirin, newer antiplatelet agents are now available. Ticlopidine was an effective alternative, but side-effects such as skin rashes and especially bone-marrow dyscrasias made its routine use unacceptable. Clopidogrel has a much better safety profile. In the CAPRIE study, clopidogrel reduced the relative risk of vascular events by 8.7% compared with aspirin.[17] Less than 1% of the patients in this study had a diagnosis of stable angina. However, clopidogrel is currently recommended for angina patients who are unable to tolerate aspirin, with a long-term prognostic benefit that is slightly superior to that of aspirin.

Lipid-lowering therapy

In general, lack of compliance with lipid-lowering diets renders them ineffective, and dyslipidaemia often warrants drug therapy. The goal of treatment is to reduce total cholesterol levels to below 5.0 mmol/L and low-density-lipoprotein (LDL) cholesterol levels to below 3.0 mmol/L. In patients with high-density-lipoprotein (HDL) cholesterol levels below 1.0 mmol/L and triglyceride levels above 2.0 mmol/L, there is an increased risk of coronary events. The choice of lipid-lowering therapy depends on the lipid profile. Serial blood lipid profiles are required to confirm the benefits of therapy. Failure to improve within 6 weeks merits a dose increase, and after 3 months it warrants a drug change or combination therapy. In patients in whom it is difficult to decrease the cholesterol level despite treatment with effective high-dose statins, referral to a specialized lipid clinic should be considered.

Statin therapy

Mechanism of action

Statins increase the number of LDL-receptors by inhibiting the enzyme HMG CoA (3-hydroxyl-3-methylglutaryl coenzyme A) reductase and so reducing total cholesterol levels. In addition, statins appear to improve endothelial dysfunction and stabilize platelet function, and may decrease fibrinogen levels.[18]

Clinical effects

Statin therapy is well established as the optimal treatment for lowering cholesterol levels in angina patients. In the 4S study, angina patients who were treated with *simvastatin* showed mortality reduced by 30%, coronary events reduced by 34% and the need for coronary revascularization reduced by 37%.[19] There was also a reduction in stroke incidence. In angina patients, statin therapy with simvastatin 20 mg daily slows disease progression in diffuse and focal coronary artery disease, and this may subsequently reduce the need for revascularization (MAAS).[20] Trials with *pravastatin* show a similar reduction in cardiac events, regression of coronary atheroma and reduction in myocardial ischaemia in angina patients on optimal anti-anginal therapy (REGRESS, PLAC1, II, LIPID).[21–23] In post-MI patients, *atorvastatin* has been shown to reduce subsequent ischaemic events, with a significant reduction in angina post MI and hospitalizations (MIRACL).[24] The benefits of statin therapy appear to be comparable across all agents in terms of event reduction and clinical benefit. However, atorvastatin produces a significantly greater reduction in LDL-cholesterol levels than do other agents (CURVES).[25]

All statins are safe and well tolerated. A recent 8-year follow-up has shown no increase in cancer deaths among these patients, and at the same duration of follow-up the clinical benefit of simvastatin was still maintained. *Fluvastatin* has a well-established role in primary and secondary prevention, and has beneficial effects on the fibrinolytic system. Novel 'superstatins' such as rosuvastatin are currently undergoing phase II trials and promise even greater lowering of LDL-cholesterol levels. Clinical data are awaited.

Alternative lipid-lowering therapies, such as bile-acid-sequestering agents (cholestyramine), nicotinic acid and fibrates, have not been evaluated in chronic stable angina patients. Although these treatments reduce cholesterol levels and in some cases help to regress coronary disease progression, their effect on cardiac mortality and morbidity in angina is unclear.

Hypertension

Rigid control is optimal. Drug therapy for hypertension can involve agents with anti-ischaemic effects that will minimize polypharmacy and improve compliance. The aim of treatment should be to lower blood pressure to below 140/85 mmHg (HOT).[26]

Diabetes mellitus

The aim of treatment is to keep the HbA_{1C} value at the lowest level (below 8) possible. In diabetic patients, it is equally important to control all risk factors for coronary artery disease in addition to blood glucose levels. The recent UK-PDS study has shown that blood pressure maintained below 150/85 mmHg and blood glucose levels maintained below 6.0 mmol/L were associated with a reduction in the risk of diabetes-related mortality and morbidity in hypertensive patients with type 2 diabetes mellitus.[27]

Hormone replacement therapy (HRT)

Women with angina who are already taking HRT can continue to do so. Patients with newly diagnosed angina or a recent MI should not be commenced on HRT, as this may increase the risk of MI and unstable angina by 33%, especially during the first year.[28] As yet there is no evidence to suggest that HRT is beneficial in the secondary prevention of coronary artery disease.

MEDICAL THERAPY FOR RELIEF OF SYMPTOMS

The choice of suitable anti-anginal treatment should consider the ischaemic mechanism of angina, the method of drug action, convenience, the cost of drug administration, drug side-effects, the usefulness of the drug for treating other conditions, contraindications to certain anti-anginal treatments, and patient compliance.

Nitrates

Mechanism of action

Nitrates reduce myocardial oxygen demand and preload, and lower LV filling pressure, intraventricular volumes and venous return.[29] At higher doses they cause arterial vasodilatation and reduce systemic vascular resistance and blood pressure, thereby relieving myocardial oxygen demand. Nitrates reduce myocardial ischaemia, relieve pain and improve exercise tolerance. However, 50% of patients may develop nitrate tolerance with continuing treatment.

The nitrate patch is best applied 12 h on and 12 h off. Unfortunately, a rebound of angina can occur during the 'off' period. This is not helped by the reflex tachycardia that may accompany the blood-pressure-reducing effect of nitrates. The tachycardia can be attenuated by concurrent beta-blockade, and any rebound angina during the nitrate-free interval can be relieved by additional anti-anginal therapy. Around 20–30% of patients on nitrate treatment experience headaches, which may necessitate reducing the drug dose or discontinuing treatment altogether.

Nitrates may be administered orally, transdermally, sublingually, buccally or as a spray. All patients, but especially those who have infrequent symptoms, should be cautioned that oral nitrates expire after 3 months.

Clinical effects

Nitrate therapy is indicated for angina that responds to sublingual glyceryl tri-nitrate (GTN). It is not recommended as first-line therapy in post-MI or hypertensive angina, except for symptom relief. Despite the absence of any prognostic data, nitrates provide excellent immediate symptomatic relief, and long-acting isosorbide mononitrate is effective with once-daily dosing.[30] If nitrate therapy is ineffective, it should be substituted with an alternative anti-anginal treatment.

Beta-blockers

Mechanism of action

Beta-blockers are highly specific competitive antagonists of the beta-receptor at its adrenergic site. They reduce myocardial oxygen demand by reducing heart rate, contractility and LV afterload, with a reduction in blood pressure at rest and on exercise (see Figure 9.2). This is achieved by blocking the cardiac beta-receptors, thus inhibiting the sinus node, atrioventricular node and myocardial contraction. It is the bradycardiac and negative inotropic effects that reduce myocardial oxygen demand. About 20% of patients do not respond to beta-blockers because they have:

1. severe obstructive coronary disease responsible for angina at a low level of exercise;

Figure 9.2
Mechanism of action of beta-blockers in angina pectoris.

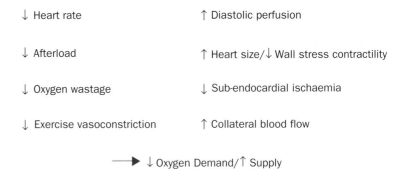

↓ Heart rate   ↑ Diastolic perfusion

↓ Afterload   ↑ Heart size/↓ Wall stress contractility

↓ Oxygen wastage   ↓ Sub-endocardial ischaemia

↓ Exercise vasoconstriction   ↑ Collateral blood flow

⟶ ↓ Oxygen Demand/↑ Supply

2. an abnormal increase in LV end-diastolic pressure resulting from an excess negative inotropic effect and a resultant decrease in sub-endocardial blood flow.

It is conventional to lower heart rates below 60 beats/min, provided that heart block does not occur and there are no symptoms. This reduced heart rate reflects persistent vagal tone at rest that accompanies the decrease in adrenergic effects. A major benefit of this is the limitation of increases in heart rate during exercise, which ideally should not increase above 100 beats/min in patients with angina. Beta-blockers are contraindicated in asthma, severe bradycardia and hypotension.

Clinical effects

Beta-blockers are particularly beneficial following MI (metoprolol reduces post-MI mortality by 36%).[31] Despite the absence of prognostic data for angina patients, the Beta-blocker Pooling Project has shown a trend towards reduced mortality in MI patients with a prior history of angina.[32] When beta-blockers need to be withdrawn, this should be done gradually, as a sudden withdrawal may up-regulate the beta-receptor and aggravate angina symptoms. Beta-blockers should be considered in angina patients with a recent MI, a history of supraventricular tachycardia, exertion-induced angina, ventricular arrhythmias or hypertension. Optimal treatment is achieved by lowering the heart rate below 50 beats/min, alleviating symptoms when there are no side-effects, and there is a blunting of the heart rate and blood pressure response to exercise. Symptomatic angina relief is established with *metoprolol, atenolol* and *propranolol* (TIBET, ASIST, APSIS, TIBBS).[33–36] *Carvedilol* is a beta-blocker with cardiac and vascular activity that reduces myocardial oxygen demand, increases blood supply and scavenges free radicals. It is as effective as other anti-anginal treatments, and may be better tolerated in patients with peripheral vascular disease and in those with LV dysfunction.[37] The latter group may also tolerate *bisoprolol* or *metoprolol slow-release* (CIBIS-II, MERIT).[38,39]

Calcium antagonists

Mechanism of action

Calcium antagonists reduce myocardial oxygen demand, afterload and heart rate, which may produce coronary artery and smooth muscle vasodilatation. In addition, they may improve blood viscosity, giving tissue protection during ischaemia, and they may even prevent the formation of new atherosclerotic lesions.[40]

Clinical effects

Dihydropyridines

Nifedipine causes peripheral vasodilatation and reflex tachycardia (which may exacerbate angina), flushing and ankle oedema. It is safest in the long-acting form, as short-acting nifedipine has been reported to increase mortality in hypertensive angina and in post-MI patients (SPRINT).[41] Nifedipine is the subject of a long-term mortality study currently ongoing in angina patients (ACTION).[40] However, it should be avoided in patients with angina due to moderate aortic stenosis or hypertrophic obstructive cardiomyopathy (HOCM). *Amlodipine* has a longer half-life and significantly reduces the frequency of pain and the need to take GTN, but it causes more ankle oedema (CAPE).[42] It is as effective as *felodipine*, and is better tolerated than diltiazem, with the added benefit of being inherently long acting. Reflex increases in heart rate can be minimized if dihydropyridines are combined with beta-blockers.

Benzothiazepines

Diltiazem reduces the heart rate and causes moderate vasodilatation. It may cause a rash, and it can increase hepatic drug levels (e.g. phenytoin). The twice-daily dose improves compliance. Diltiazem reduces reinfarction in MI patients, and should be considered for angina patients who cannot take beta-blockers.[43]

Phenylalkylamines

Verapamil reduces heart rate and blood pressure. It may cause constipation and intense bradycardia. Caution is needed in patients with LV dysfunction and in Wolff–Parkinson–White syndrome, where verapamil should be avoided. Verapamil reduces cardiac events and angina post MI (DAVIT),[44] especially when beta-blockers were not used. The sustained-release once-daily dose is well tolerated, very effective and improves compliance. Like diltiazem, no mortality data are available for verapamil in angina patients. Calcium-channel blockers should be considered in angina patients if beta-blockers are contraindicated, and in vasospastic angina.

Trimetazidine (Vastarel)

Conventional anti-anginal therapy works by reducing oxygen demand or enhancing delivery. An alternative approach is to modify the consequences of ischaemia at the cellular level. Pharmacological optimization of cardiac metabolism without causing any direct haemodynamic, inotropic and chronotropic effects may be particularly useful when treating angina patients. Trimetazidine is a cellular anti-ischaemic agent that enhances glucose oxidation and provides myocardial cytoprotection. It improves cardiac work, exercise tolerance and time to ST-segment depression without changing heart rate and blood pressure.[45] It is effective either as monotherapy or as combination therapy with a beta-blocker or diltiazem. Its side-effect profile is excellent.

Nicorandil

This is a potassium-channel opener with nitrate-like vasodilating properties.[46] It provides myocardial cytoprotection and reduces ischaemia. It is effective as monotherapy in patients with minimal exertional symptoms. Headaches may require the dose to be titrated gradually. There is now more information about nicorandil as combination therapy, but it does have a significant nitrate-like effect and may therefore have an important role in treating high-risk stable angina patients. The recent Impact of Nicorandil in Angina (IONA) trial, assessing the effect of nicorandil on cardiovascular events in a stable population, showed a significant improvement in clinical outcome after 18 months.[46]

Monotherapy or combined therapy for symptom relief? (Box 9.4)

Monotherapy studies have failed to show a consistent advantage of one treatment over another. Effective anti-anginal treatment is probably best served by beta-blockers or calcium-channel blockers, in view of tolerance problems with nitrates. All patients should be offered short-acting nitrates either by spray or sublingually for symptom relief and for prophylactic use (e.g. prior to exercise). Cardioselective beta-blockers are preferred, except for angina patients with ventricular arrhythmias, for whom sotalol may be preferred, or for thyrotoxic angina patients, for whom propranolol may be used. Ideally, a long-acting beta-blocker will improve compliance, especially when stopping treatment suddenly may exacerbate symptoms. Calcium antagonists are advised if beta-blockers are contraindicated, and for coronary artery spasm, hypertension, diabetes, peripheral vascular disease, bronchospasm and Raynaud's phenomenon. Diltiazem and verapamil are equally effective. Amlodipine may improve compliance. Monotherapy should involve switching from one agent to another if it is ineffective, before switching to combination therapy.

Combination therapy may reduce side-effects, offset the side-effects of monotherapy, or provide longer anti-anginal cover, but equally it may exacerbate hypotension and bradycardia, worsening perfusion or precipitating heart failure, and it may even antagonize the therapeutic effect of monotherapy. It is more expensive, compliance is poorer, and combinations such as beta-blockers and verapamil may cause heart block and other adverse effects. However, combination therapy (two or three drugs) may be needed to control

---

Box 9.4   Drug therapy for stable angina pectoris: symptom control

Beta-blockers
  Atenolol, 25–100 mg daily
  Bisoprolol, 5–20 mg
  Carvedilol, 12.5–25 mg
    twice a day
  Metoprolol, 50–100 mg
    three times a day
  Nadolol, 40–160 mg
  Propranolol, 40–80 mg
    three times a day
  Oxyprenolol, 80–320 mg
    three times a day
  Timolol, 5–15 mg
    three times a day
Calcium antagonists
  Amlodipine, 5–10 mg
  Diltiazem, 60–120 mg
    three times a day
    (slow release preferred)
  Nifedipine, 20–40 mg
    (slow release preferred)
  Verapamil, 80–120 mg
    three times a day
    (slow release preferred)
  Felodipine, 5–10 mg

Nitrates (sublingual
transdermal, oral)
  Isosorbide mononitrate,
    10–40 mg three times a day
  Isosorbide dinitrate,
    30–240 mg daily
  Transdermal patch,
    5–20 mg daily
Trimetazidine
  (Vastarel) 20 mg three
    times a day
Nicorandil
  10–20 mg twice a day

---

more severe symptoms, especially if revascularization is not an option (30% of patients). Effective combinations include nitrate and beta-blockers (metoprolol). Calcium-channel blockers and nitrates are useful for spasm. Calcium-channel blockers and beta-blockers will reduce side-effects and dose. Nifedipine, amlodipine and felodipine have all been shown to improve symptoms when combined with beta-blockers (FEMINA),[47] in some cases more than taking beta-blockers alone (CAPE).[42] Around 10–15% of patients who are taking a beta-blocker and verapamil may experience significant bradycardia, heart block, hypotension and heart failure. Calcium antagonists and nitrates may not provide additive anti-anginal effects. Triple therapy, although widely used, is of doubtful benefit to the patient. Those patients who continue to have poorly controlled symptoms should be referred for angiography. As metabolic agents differ from conventional anti-anginal treatment in their mechanism of action, the combination of metabolic and haemodynamic therapy is an alternative approach in patients who are not adequately controlled on monotherapy.

Adjunctive therapy

ACE inhibitors

ACE inhibitors reduce ischaemic events in MI patients (SAVE, SOLVD, AIRE)[48–50] with LV dysfunction. In patients with coronary artery disease who have normal LV function, the HOPE study has shown that ramipril reduces the risk of MI by 22%, reduces the risk of stroke by 32%, and reduces the risk of cardiovascular death by 26%.[51] This benefit is in part due to a regression in atherosclerosis (SECURE),[52] and may also be due to an effect on endothelial dysfunction (TREND).[53] Further ACE-inhibitor studies (i.e. EUROPA, PEACE)[54] are evaluating ACE-inhibitor therapy in similar patient groups with normal LV systolic function.

Vitamin supplements

The role of vitamin therapy in cardiovascular disease is based on preventing the oxidation of LDL, mitigating the adverse effects of the scavenger pathway and ultimately preventing atherosclerosis at an early stage. Significant risk reductions (50%) in the prevalence of coronary artery disease have been observed in individuals with a high intake of foods rich in vitamin E. Among patients with angina/angiographic evidence of coronary artery disease, three randomized controlled trials have been reported. The CHAOS study in the UK found that alpha-tocopherol reduced the risk of non-fatal MI or cardiac death by 47%. There was a 77% reduction in non-fatal MI. However, there was an 18% increased risk of fatal MI. The clinical benefit within the CHAOS study may have been due to a selected population with a high genetic predisposition to reduced endothelial function that was particularly susceptible to the beneficial effects of vitamin E.[55] The ATBC trial involving Finnish smokers, which included 1862 patients with previous MI, showed a 38% reduction in non-fatal MI in patients taking vitamin E.[56] However, like the CHAOS group, there was an increase in fatal MI and also in haemorrhagic stroke (which may have been due to an adverse effect on the coagulation cascade). The ATBC trial was terminated early because of this. In patients who received vitamins C and E there was also an increase in mortality. The GISSI prevention trial also failed to show any benefit of taking vitamin E post MI.[57] In the HOPE study, the addition of vitamin E to ACE-inhibitor therapy did not confer any additional benefit in patients with coronary artery disease.[58] The current advice for stable angina patients with regard to vitamin supplements is that the evidence does not support taking supplements to improve the prognosis, but a healthy diet will often include abundant antioxidants and is strongly recommended for secondary prevention.

Intervention-based treatment of chronic stable angina

CORONARY ANGIOGRAPHY

This is the gold standard for diagnosing coronary artery disease. Coronary angiography is indicated in patients with severe chronic stable angina that is not responding to medical treatment, with chronic stable angina with low exercise tolerance, with chronic stable angina with bundle branch block, with reversible ischaemia on perfusion scan, with angina with serious ventricular arrhythmias, or with recurrent angina following coronary artery bypass graft (CABG) or angioplasty, and in some preoperative situations (e.g. before surgery for abdominal aortic aneurysm/carotid disease in patients with angina). In cases where the diagnosis of angina is likely to have a significant effect on the patient's livelihood (e.g. airline pilot), coronary angiography is also indicated. Although angiography only gives a two-dimensional image of the vessel lumen, a normal study is immensely reassuring.

REVASCULARIZATION

In general, revascularization is performed either to relieve intractable symptoms (CABG or angioplasty) or to improve a poor prognosis (CABG).

Coronary angioplasty (percutaneous coronary angioplasty) with or without stenting

This provides symptom relief, reduces the need to take medication, and improves exercise performance and quality of life. In stable angina, percutaneous coronary angioplasty (PTCA) is successful in 95% of cases (see Figure 9.3). The mortality rate is 0.2–0.5%, depending on whether there is single-vessel or multi-vessel disease. Less than 1% of cases will require emergency CABG. The rate of procedural MI is also less than 1%. The procedure is quick and hospitalization is short, allowing a rapid return to work. Unfortunately, 15–30% of cases restenose, and this may be asymptomatic. Exercise testing is poorly predictive of this, but good exercise tolerance confers a good prognosis. The introduction of stenting, and the recent arrival of anti-proliferative drug eluting stents, has significantly reduced the risk of restenosis. The BENESTENT study showed that stenting reduced the need for repeat revascularization, compared with angioplasty.[59] The follow-on study, BENESTENT II,[60] confirmed that stents were superior to angioplasty, and the STRESS[61] study confirmed that stenting reduces 6-month restenosis and the need for revascularization. In angina patients with chronic occlusions, stenting improves the short-term results compared with angioplasty, and also reduces major cardiac events (SICCO).[62]

Figure 9.3
Stent after coronary artery bypass graft (CABG). Coronary angioplasty and stent placement in a left internal mammary artery (LIMA) graft as it anastomoses with the native left anterior descending artery (LADA). A tight stenosis (a) is treated by inflating balloon and stent (b), with excellent angiographic results (c).

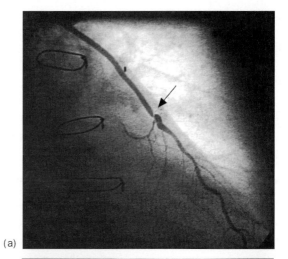
(a)

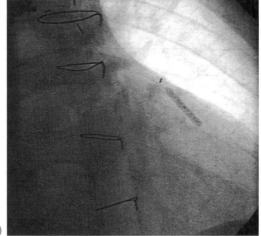
(b)

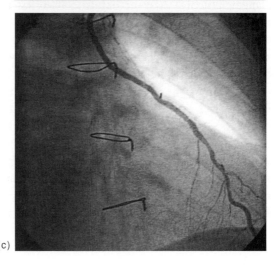
(c)

Other percutaneous devices that have been introduced as alternatives to balloon angioplasty, including laser, directional atherectomy, rotational atherectomy, cutting and suction devices, have found no specific role in general percutaneous coronary intervention practice (CAVEAT-1, CAVEAT-II [atherectomy], AMRO [laser], ERBAC [laser plus atherectomy], BOAT [atherectomy], MUSIC [intravascular ultrasound], START [stent vs. intravascular ultrasound (IVUS) plus atherectomy]).[63-69] If applied, these devices are often used as an adjunct to balloon angioplasty, and are only occasionally used as a stand-alone procedure.

There is no evidence pointing to the superiority of PTCA over medical therapy in terms of infarction or mortality in patients with stable angina. The ACME, RITA-2 and AVERT trials have demonstrated in selected stable angina patients (ACME, one-vessel disease and mild angina; RITA-2, one-vessel or two-vessel disease and mild to moderate angina; AVERT, mildly symptomatic and one-vessel disease)[70-72] that medical treatment was only slightly less efficacious in alleviating symptoms and improving exercise tolerance than angioplasty, whilst the prognosis was comparable in both groups. These studies suggest and reconfirm that an initial medical treatment strategy should be attempted to relieve or control anginal symptoms in patients with mild stable angina. If this should fail, revascularization is recommended. In the ACME study, angioplasty for single-vessel disease improved symptoms and normalized exercise tolerance,[70] but PTCA was expensive and had higher complication rates. Angioplasty should be considered for single-vessel disease and multi-vessel disease, and for patients with symptoms that are not controlled by medical therapy. Patients with single-vessel disease derive no prognostic benefit from CABG. Ongoing advances in stenting (coated stents),[73] antiplatelet therapy (glycoprotein IIb/IIIa receptor antagonists),[74,75] adjunctive medical therapy (diltiazem, probucol, thromboxane A_2 antagonists)[76-78] and newer technology (laser–brachytherapy)[79] should help to reduce PTCA restenosis and make PTCA a more effective therapy for patients with chronic stable angina. Long-term follow up with coated stents (RAVEL)[73] is eagerly awaited and may revolutionize the approach to coronary intervention.

Coronary artery bypass grafting surgery (CABG)
CABG has been shown to improve the prognosis in angina patients with the following:

- left main stem stenosis;
- three-vessel disease with LV dysfunction;
- three-vessel disease with moderate/severe symptoms or an early positive exercise test;
- two-vessel disease where one vessel involves the proximal left anterior descending artery;
- (in high-risk patients) positive early non-invasive tests at low workloads.

High-risk patients (older patients and those with LV dysfunction, more severe disease, more severe proximal stenoses threatening larger amounts of heart muscle, or renal and respiratory comorbidity, diabetics, and female patients with multi-vessel disease) are likely to benefit most from CABG. The complication rates are higher, with an in-hospital mortality rate of 4–5% and perioperative MI rate of 4–5%. Therefore high-risk patients have more to gain but are at greater risk during CABG, which means that the decision as to whether to perform CABG in such a patient requires full discussion of the individual case with the patient, the cardiologist and the surgeon.

The choice of surgery vs. PTCA in stable angina has been addressed in a number of multicentre trials (RITA-1, ERAC-I, GABI, EAST, CABRI, BARI and ARTS).[80–86] In summary, angioplasty and CABG perform equally well, but patients undergoing the former have tended to show a greater recurrence of angina and the need for repeat PTCA or CABG. In the EAST and BARI studies, comparing PTCA and CABG in multi-vessel disease, the need for revascularization was increased up to 3 years after the initial PTCA, but at 5-year follow-up in BARI, the benefit of both interventions was the same, making PTCA a more cost-effective treatment for angina patients.[83,85] As has already been mentioned, certain subgroups of patients (female patients with multi-vessel disease, and diabetics) had an improved prognosis with initial CABG rather than PTCA, especially if arterial grafts had been used. An interesting finding from the ARTS study was that state-of-the-art stenting reduced the need for repeat procedures or revascularization from 25% to 13%.[86] The benefit of stenting over PTCA alone is clear, and compared with CABG in angina patients it is currently under evaluation in the BARI-2 study.

CABG with arterial grafting using both internal mammary arteries and the radial artery gives greater symptomatic relief and long-term patency (90% of left internal mammary artery grafts are patent at 10 years). Newer surgical procedures (e.g. a minimally invasive approach via a small thoracotomy to the beating heart without the use of cardiopulmonary bypass, thereby avoiding its associated cerebral complications) are nowadays safe and feasible, but only for certain well-defined anatomical bypasses. This less invasive approach is unquestionably more attractive to patients. Its definitive place is currently being determined by the Octopus trial, which is comparing minimally invasive direct coronary artery bypass (MIDCAB) with stent implantation.[87]

Repeat CABG carries a high risk, depending on LV function, with a 5–11% mortality rate. Compared with medical therapy, CABG reduces mortality in high-risk groups. In comparison with angioplasty, both CABG and PTCA have a similar risk of mortality and fatal MI. CABG causes longer hospitalization, as well as exposure to infection, major surgery and longer recovery, but patients often have less angina, requiring fewer medications. PTCA is quick, can be performed as a day case, and has a short recovery time, but some patients, particularly women, have more angina, requiring more medication and often CABG.

In the long term, PTCA may be more cost-effective and a lower-risk procedure compared with redoing CABG, but long-term data are not available.

Current position with regard to PTCA vs. CABG: unresolved questions

Angioplasty with stenting is the preferred strategy for single-vessel disease. It is also preferred for multi-vessel disease if the lesions are suitable for percutaneous interventions. Surgery is preferred for left main stem disease and multi-vessel disease that is not amenable to PTCA. All significant lesions supplying viable myocardium should be treated. There are still unresolved issues regarding the optimal treatment strategy. These issues pertain to lesion size, length, chronic occlusions, vein graft stenosis, left main stem lesions and bifurcation lesions, as well as clinical comorbidities such as diabetes mellitus and advancing age (especially over 75 years). These issues are all undergoing evaluation in clinical trials, and until they have been resolved, consensus between cardiologists and surgeons should determine the optimal treatment strategy for the individual patient.

EMERGING THERAPIES FOR STABLE ANGINA PATIENTS
(see Box 9.5)

External body counter-pulsation

This therapy involves wrapping inflatable cuffs around the patient's legs. The cuffs are inflated with compressed air in a sequence that is synchronized with the cardiac cycle. The technique increases retrograde aortic blood flow during diastole and decreases vascular impedance. The device is commercially available.

The clinical benefit of enhanced external counter-pulsation is validated by the MUST-EECP study, in which stable angina patients with class I–III angina and documented coronary artery disease plus a positive exercise test underwent 4–7 weeks of such treatment.[88] These patients showed decreased angina frequency and improved time to exercise-induced ischaemia. There was also a trend towards a reduction in GTN use.

Box 9.5   Novel therapies for refractive angina

- External body counter-pulsation
- Spinal cord stimulators
- Destructive sympathectomies
- TMR/PMR

Spinal cord stimulators (SCS)

For patients with intractable angina who are on maximal medical treatment and unsuitable for intervention, new devices known as spinal cord stimulators have been developed to reduce symptoms. Clinical evidence supporting the use of SCS comes from the Electrical Stimulation Bypass Surgery (ESBY) study comparing SCS with CABG in patients who are unsuitable for angioplasty. In this case, SCS implantation led to a reduction in angina symptoms and increased exercise capacity.[89] In selected patients, SCS may be a useful adjunctive anti-anginal therapy.

Destructive sympathectomy

Sympathectomy involves destruction of the sympathetic fibres that innervate the heart. This can be achieved by chemical methods (alcohol injection of the upper four thoracic ganglia), surgery or thoracoscopic methods. Chemical sympathectomy has lost favour as a consequence of improved anaesthesia and reduced surgical mortality rates. Thoracoscopic sympathectomy has been reported in intractable angina patients who were unsuitable for surgery due to a high operative risk or unsuitable coronary anatomy. In Claes' series of 43 patients, all of the study subjects showed significant reductions in the number of angina attacks and use of GTN at 4–7 weeks after sympathectomy, and 19 patients were free of angina symptoms at 1 year.[90] These patients also showed improved exercise capacity, as has been verified by Khogali *et al.* in another study of similar patients treated with thoracoscopic sympathectomy for intractable angina.[91]

Transmyocardial laser revascularization (TMR)

TMR burns multiple small channels into the myocardium. It can lead to a reduction in angina symptoms as well as to improved exercise tolerance. Unfortunately, all TMR studies have found an increase in mortality rate associated with this form of treatment. This increase in mortality was especially marked in patients with a left ventricular ejection fraction (LVEF) of $< 40\%$. The recent ATLANTIC study of TMR showed that the latter was superior to medical therapy and improved exercise tolerance in intractable angina patients on maximum medical therapy, but despite this clinical effect, no evidence of improved myocardial perfusion was found on thallium perfusion scans.[92] Use of a CO_2 laser with TMR has shown symptomatic improvement in angina symptoms, but no improvement in exercise tolerance.[93] Although TMR requires open-heart surgery, a percutaneous approach (percutaneous myocardial revascularization or PMR) (i.e. catheter based) is also available. In the PACIFIC trial, PMR with an yttrium–aluminium–garnet laser was assessed in angina patients.[94] Patients reported an improvement in angina symptoms and in exercise tolerance, and the procedure was well tolerated. There may be a place for TMR or PMR as an alternative anti-anginal therapy in cases where no other treatment options exist. There is unquestionably a significant placebo effect, and disagreement about the basic mechanism of benefit is a disturbing reminder that the technique is still in its infancy.

Conclusions

The management of stable angina pectoris aims to improve symptoms and to try to improve the prognosis. The general steps of identifying and treating risk factors are paramount. These include smoking cessation, diet, exercise and lifestyle modification. Aspirin and lipid-lowering agents should probably be given to all patients.

Medical therapy with a beta-blocker is advised unless it is contraindicated. Otherwise a calcium antagonist, nitrate, nicorandil or trimetazidine should be taken. GTN spray should be used for short-term relief.

In high-risk patients, early angiography may be appropriate, with or without revascularization; otherwise, medical therapy should be intensified. If the symptoms do not settle, then revascularization should be performed as follows:

1. PTCA plus stenting for single-vessel and multi-vessel disease;
2. CABG for left main stem disease and multi-vessel disease that is not suitable for PTCA.

In women with multi-vessel disease, diabetics and patients with LV systolic dysfunction, CABG may be the preferred treatment. Secondary prevention, especially lipid-lowering therapy and smoking cessation, will influence the outcome of revascularization in terms of success as well as graft patency. In patients who are unsuitable for CABG/PTCA, new therapies such as PMR, external body counter-pulsation and SCS may be considered for intractable symptoms.

Many unanswered questions still remain with regard to defining the ideal treatment approach, and until these dilemmas have been resolved by ongoing clinical trials, a consensus between cardiologist and surgeon is required when treating each individual patient. The enormous advances of medical therapy and coronary artery intervention have transformed the current management of patients with chronic stable angina, not only in terms of relieving symptoms, but also by improving their prognosis.

References

1. DeBono A. *The investigation and management of stable angina. Report of the Joint Audit Committee of the British Cardiac Society and Royal*

College of Physicians. London: British Cardiac Society and Royal College of Surgeons, 1996.

2. Task Force of the European Society of Cardiology. Guidelines. The management of stable angina pectoris. *Eur Heart J* 1997; **18**: 394–413.

3. Task Force of the European Society of Cardiology. Guidelines. Prevention of coronary artery disease in clinical practice. *Eur Heart J* 1998; **19**: 1434–503.

4. North of England Evidence-Based Guideline Development Project. The primary care management of stable angina. Evidence-based clinical practice guidelines. *Br Med J* 1996; **312**: 827–32.

5. Solomon AJ, Gersh B. Management of chronic stable angina: medical therapy, PTCA and CABG. *Ann Intern Med* 1998; **128**: 216–23.

6. Jorenby DE, Leischow SJ, Nides MA *et al.* A controlled trial of sustained-release bupropion, a nicotine patch or both for smoking cessation. *N Engl J Med* 1999; **340**: 685–91.

7. de Lorgeil M, Salen P, Martia JL *et al.* Lyon Diet Heart Study: Mediterranean diet, traditional risk factors and rate of cardiovascular complications after myocardial infarction. *Circulation* 1999; **99**: 779–85.

8. UK Guidelines on Driving; www.dvla.gov.uk@_a_glance/ch2_cardiovascular.htm

9. Shakir SA, Wilton LV, Boshier A *et al.* Cardiovascular events in users of sildenafil: results from the first phase of prescription event monitoring in England. *Br Med J* 2001; **322**: 651–2.

10. Opie LH. *Drugs for the heart*, 4th edn. New York: WB Saunders, 1995.

11. Hjemdahl P, Eriksson SV, Held C *et al.* Prognosis of patients with stable angina pectoris on antianginal drug therapy. *Am J Cardiol* 1996; **77**: 6–15D.

12. Parker JD. Clinical outcome studies of antianginal drug therapy for patients with stable coronary artery disease: an indication for clinical trials. *Eur Heart J* 1998; **19 (Supplement I)**: 115–19.

13. Fuster V, Dyken ML, Vokonas PS, Hennekens C. Aspirin as a therapeutic agent in cardiovascular disease. *Circulation* 1993; **87**: 659–75.

14. Juul-Moller S, Edvardson N, Jahnmatz B *et al.* for the SAPAT (Swedish Angina Pectoris Aspirin Trial) Group. Double-blind trial of aspirin in primary prevention of myocardial infarction in patients with stable angina pectoris. *Lancet* 1992; **340**: 1421–5.

15. Ridker PM, Manson JE, Gaziano M *et al.* Low-dose aspirin therapy for chronic stable angina. A randomised, placebo-controlled trial. *Ann Intern Med* 1991; **114**: 835–9.

16. ISIS-2 Collaborators. International Study of Infarct Survival 2. *Lancet* 1988; **ii**: 349–60.

17. CAPRIE Steering Committee. A randomised, blinded trial of clopidogrel versus aspirin in patients at risk of ischaemic events (CAPRIE). *Lancet* 1996; **348**: 1329–39.

18. Koh KK. Effects of statins on vascular wall: vasomotor function, inflammation and plaque stability. *Cardiovasc Res* 2000; **47**: 648–57.

19. Scandinavian Simvastatin Survival Study Group. Randomised trial of cholesterol lowering in 4444 patients with coronary artery disease. 4S Study. *Lancet* 1994; **344**: 1383–9.

20. MAAS Investigators. Effect of simvastatin on coronary atheroma: the Multicentre Anti-Atheroma Study (MAAS). *Lancet* 1994; **344**: 633–8.

21. Van Boven AJ, Jukema JW, Zwinderman AH *et al.* Reduction of transient myocardial ischaemia with pravastatin in addition to the conventional treatment in patients with angina pectoris. *Circulation* 1996; **94**: 1503–5.

22. Furberg CD, Pitt B, Byington RP *et al.* Pravastatin limitation of athero-sclerosis in the coronary arteries. *Am J Cardiol* 1995; **76**: 60–3C.

23. The LIPID Study Group. Prevention of cardiovascular events and death with pravastatin in patients with coronary heart disease. *N Engl J Med* 1998; **339**: 1349–57.

24. Schwartz GG, Olson AG, Ezekowitz MD *et al.* Effects of atorvastatin on early recurrent ischaemic events in acute coronary syndromes: MIRACL Study. *J Am Med Assoc* 2001; **285**: 1711–18.

25. Jones P, Kafonek S, Laurora I *et al.* Comparative dose efficacy of ator-vastatin, simvastatin, pravastatin, lovastatin and fluvastatin in patients with hypercholesterolemia (the CURVES Study). *Am J Cardiol* 1998; **81**: 582–7.

26. Hansson L, Zanchetti A. The Hypertension Optimal Treatment (HOT) Study: 24-month data on blood pressure and tolerability. *Blood Pressure* 1997; **6**: 313–17.

27. UK Prospective Diabetes Study Group. Tight blood pressure control and risk of macrovascular and microvascular complications in type 2 diabetes mellitus. *Br Med J* 1998; **317**: 703–13.

28. Josefson D. Women with heart disease cautioned about HRT. *Br Med J* 1999; **318**: 753–4.

29. Parker JD, Parker JO. Nitrate therapy for stable angina pectoris. *N Engl J Med* 1998; **338**: 520–31.

30. Prakash A, Markham A. Long-acting isosorbide mononitrate. *Drugs* 1999; **57**: 93–9.

31. The MIAMI Research Group. Metoprolol in acute myocardial infarction – randomised placebo-controlled trial. *Eur Heart J* 1985; **6**: 199–226.

32. Beta-Blocker Pooling Project Research Group. Subgroup findings from randomised trials in post-myocardial infarction patients. *Eur Heart J* 1988; **9**: 8–16.

33. Dargie HJ, Ford I, Fox KM *et al.* for the TIBET Study Group. Total Ischaemic Burden European Trial (TIBET): effect of ischaemia and treatment with atenolol, nifedipine SR and their combination on outcome in patients with chronic stable angina. *Eur Heart J* 1996; **17**: 104–12.

34. Pepine C, Cohn PF, Deedwania PC *et al.* Effects of treatment on outcome in mildly symptomatic patients with ischaemia during daily life. The Atenolol Silent Ischaemia Study (ASIST). *Circulation* 1994; **90**: 762–8.

35. Rehnquist N, Hjemdahl P, Billing E *et al.* Effects of metoprolol versus verapamil in patients with stable angina pectoris. The Angina Prognosis Study in Stockholm (APSIS). *Eur Heart J* 1996; **17**: 76–81.

36. Von Arnim T for the Total Ischemic Burden Bisoprolol Study (TIBBS) Investigators. Total Ischaemic Burden Bisoprolol Study. *J Am Coll Cardiol* 1995; **25**: 231–8.

37. Sorelle R. Copernicus affirmed. *Circulation* 2000; **102**: E9026.

38. CIBIS-II Investigators. The Cardiac Insufficiency Bisoprolol Study II. *Lancet* 1999; **353**: 9–13.

39. Hjamarson A, Goldstein S, Fagerberg B *et al.* Metoprolol CR/XL randomized intervention trial in congestive heart failure. *J Am Med Assoc* 2000; **283**: 1295–302.

40. Silvestry FE, St John Sutton G. Sustained-release calcium-channel antagonists in cardiovascular disease: pharmacology and current therapeutic use. *Eur Heart J* 1998; **338**: 520–31.

41. Goldbourt U, Behar S, Reicher-Reiss H *et al.* Early administration of nifedipine in suspected acute myocardial infarction. *Arch Intern Med* 1993; **153**: 345–53.

42. Deanfield JE, Detry J-MRG, Lichtlen PR *et al.* Amlodipine reduces transient myocardial ischemia in patients with coronary artery disease (CAPE trial). *J Am Coll Cardiol* 1994; **24**: 1460–7.

43. The Multicenter Diltiazem Post-Infarction Trial Research Group. The effect of diltiazem on mortality and reinfarction after myocardial infarction. *N Engl J Med* 1988; **319**: 385–92.

44. DAVIT Group. The Danish Verapamil Infarction Trial. *Am J Cardiol* 1990; **66**: 779–85.

45. Szwed H, Hradec J, Preda I. Anti-ischaemic efficacy and tolerability of trimetazidine administered to patients with angina pectoris: results of three studies. *Coron Artery Dis* 2001; **12 (Supplement I)**: 525–8.

46. The IONA Study Group. Effect of nicorandil on coronary events in patients with stable angina: the Impact of Nicorandil in Angina (IONA) randomised trial. *Lancet* 2002; **359**(9314): 1269–75.

47. Dunselman P, Liem AH, Verdel G *et al.* Felodipine ER and metoprolol CR in angina (FEMINA). Working group on cardiovascular research, The Netherlands. *Eur Heart J* 1997; **18**: 1755–64.

48. Pfeffer MA, Braunwald E, Moye L *et al.* Effect of captopril on mortality and morbidity in patients with left ventricular dysfunction after myocardial infarction. Results of the Survival and Ventricular Enlargement Trial. *N Engl J Med* 1992; **327**: 669–77.

49. The SOLVD Investigators. Effect of enalapril on mortality and the development of heart failure in asymptomatic patients with reduced left ventricular ejection fraction. *N Engl J Med* 1992; **327**: 685–91.

50. The Acute Infarction Ramipril Efficacy Study Investigators. Effect of ramipril on mortality and morbidity of survivors of acute myocardial infarction with clinical evidence of heart failure. *Lancet* 1993; **342**: 821–8.

51. The HOPE Study Investigators. Effect of angiotensin-converting-enzyme inhibitor, ramipril, on cardiovascular outcomes in high-risk patients. *N Engl J Med* 2000; **342**: 145–53.

52. Lonn EM, Yusuf S, Doris CI *et al.* Study design and baseline characteristics of the study to evaluate carotid ultrasound changes in patients treated with ramipril and vitamin E: SECURE. *Am J Cardiol* 1999; **78**: 914–19.

53. Mancini GBJ, Henry GC, Macaya C *et al.* Trial on reversing endothelial dysfunction. *Circulation* 1996; **94**: 258–65.

54. Simoons ML, Vos J, de Freyter PJ *et al.* EUROPA substudies: confirmation of pathophysiological concepts. European trial on reduction of cardiac events with perindopril in stable coronary artery disease. *Eur Heart J* 1998; **19 (Supplement J)**: 56–60.

55. Stephens NG, Parsons A, Schofield PM *et al.* Randomised controlled trial of vitamin E in patients with coronary disease: Cambridge Heart Antioxidant Study (CHAOS). *Lancet* 1996; **347**: 781–6.

56. Rapola JM, Virtamo J, Ripatti S *et al.* Effects of alpha-tocopherol and beta-carotene supplements on symptoms, progression and prognosis of angina pectoris. *Heart* 1998; **79**: 454–8.

57. GISSI-Prevenzione Investigators. Dietary supplementation with n-3 polyunsaturated fatty acids and vitamin E after myocardial infarction. *Lancet* 1999; **354**: 447–55.

58. The HOPE Investigators. Vitamin E supplementation and cardiovascular events in high-risk patients. *N Engl J Med* 2000; **342**: 154–60.

59. Serruys PW, deJaegere P, Kiemenij F *et al.* A comparison of balloon-expandable stent implantation in patients with coronary artery disease. *N Engl J Med* 1994; **331**: 489–95.

60. Serruys PW, van Hout B, Bonnier H *et al.* Randomised comparison of implantation of heparin-coated stents with balloon angioplasty in selected patients with coronary artery disease. *Lancet* 1998; **352**: 673–81.

61. George CJ, Baim DS, Brinker JA *et al.* One-year follow-up of the Stent Restenosis (STRESS-1) Study. *Am J Cardiol* 1998; **81**: 860–5.

62. Sirnes PA, Golf S, Myreng Y *et al.* Sustained benefit of stenting chronic coronary occlusion: long-term follow-up of the Stenting in Chronic Coronary Occlusion (SICCO) Study. *J Am Coll Cardiol* 1998; **32**: 305–10.

63. Topol EJ, Leya F, Pinkerton CA *et al.* A comparison of directional atherectomy with coronary angioplasty in patients with coronary artery disease. *N Engl J Med* 1993; **329**: 221–7.

64. Holmes DR, Topol EJ, Califf RM *et al.* A multicenter, randomized trial of coronary angioplasty vs directional atherectomy for patients with saphenous vein bypass graft lesions. *Circulation* 1995; **91**: 1966–74.

65. Appleman YEA, Piek JJ, Strikwerda S *et al.* Randomised trial of excimer laser angioplasty vs balloon angioplasty for treatment of obstructive coronary artery disease. *Lancet* 1996; **347**: 79–84.

66. Reifart N, Vandormael M, Krajcar M *et al.* Randomized comparison of angioplasty of complex coronary lesions at a single center. Excimer Laser, Rotational Atherectomy and Balloon Angioplasty Comparison (ERBAC) Study. *Circulation* 1997; **96**: 91–8.

67. Baim DS, Cutlip DE, Sharma SK *et al.* Final results of the Balloon vs Optimal Atherectomy Trial (BOAT). *Circulation* 1998; **97**: 322–31.

68. DeJaegere P, Mudra P, Figulla H *et al.* Intravascular ultrasound-guided optimised stent deployment. *Eur Heart J* 1998; **19**: 1214–23.

69. Tsuchikane E, Sumitsujii S, Awata N *et al.* Final results of the Stent vs Directional Coronary Atherectomy Randomised Trial (START). *J Am Coll Cardiol* 1999; **34**: 1050–7.

70. Parisi AF, Folland ED, Hartigan P *et al.* A comparison of angioplasty with medical therapy in the treatment of single-vessel coronary artery disease. *N Engl J Med* 1992; **326**: 10–16.

71. RITA-2 Trial Participants. Coronary angioplasty vs medical therapy for angina: the second Randomised Intervention Treatment of Angina (RITA-2). *Lancet* 1997; **350**: 461–8.

72. Pitt B, Waters D, Brown WV *et al.* Aggressive lipid-lowering therapy compared with angioplasty in stable coronary artery disease. *N Engl J Med* 1999; **341**: 70–6.

73. Morice M-C, Serruys PW, Sousa JE *et al.* A randomized comparison of a sirolimus-eluting stent with a standard stent for coronary revascularization. RAVEL. *N Engl J Med* 2002; **346**: 1773–80.

74. Mehta SR, Yusuf S. The Clopidogrel in Unstable Angina to Prevent Recurrent Events (CURE) trial programme. *Eur Heart J* 2000; **21**: 2033–41.

75. The EPILOG Investigators. Platelet glycoprotein 2B/3A receptor blockade and low-dose heparin during percutaneous coronary revascularization. *N Engl J Med* 1997; **336**: 1689–96.

76. Lablanche J-M, Grollier G, Lusson J-R *et al.* Effect of the direct nitric oxide donors linsidomine and molsidomine on angiographic restenosis after coronary balloon angioplasty. The ACCORD study. *Circulation* 1997; **95**: 83–9.

77. Tardif J-C, Cote G, Lesperance J *et al.* Probucol and multivitamins in the prevention of restenosis after coronary angioplasty. *N Engl J Med* 1997; **337**: 365–72.

78. Savage MP, Goldberg S, Bove AA *et al.* Effect of thromboxane A$_2$ blockade on clinical outcome and restenosis after successful coronary angioplasty. Multi-Hospital Eastern Atlantic Restenosis trial (M-HEART II). *Circulation* 1995; **92**: 3194–200.

79. Waksman R, White L, Chan RC *et al.* Intracoronary gamma radiation after angioplasty inhibits reccurrence in patients with in-stent restenosis. *Circulation* 2000; **101**: 2165–71.

80. RITA Trial Participants. Coronary angioplasty vs coronary artery bypass surgery: the Randomised Intervention Treatment of Angina (RITA) trial. *Lancet* 1993; **341**: 573–80.

81. Rodriguez A, Buollon F, Perez-Balino N *et al.* Argentine randomized trial of percutaneous transluminal coronary angioplasty vs coronary artery bypass surgery in multivessel disease (ERAC 1). *J Am Coll Cardiol* 1993; **22**: 1060–7.

82. Hamm CW, Reimers J, Ischinger T *et al.* A randomized study of coronary angioplasty compared with bypass surgery in patients with symptomatic multivessel coronary disease. *N Engl J Med* 1994; **331**: 1037–43.

83. King SB III, Lembo NJ, Weintraub WS *et al.* A randomized trial comparing coronary angioplasty with bypass surgery. *N Engl J Med* 1994; **331**: 1044–50.

84. CABRI Trial Investigators. First-year results of CABRI (Coronary Angioplasty vs Bypass Revascularisation Investigation). *Lancet* 1995; **346**: 1179–84.

85. The BARI Investigators. Comparison of coronary artery bypass surgery with angioplasty in patients with multivessel disease. *N Engl J Med* 1996; **335**: 217–25.

86. ARTS Study Group. Comparison of CABG and stenting for treatment of multivessel disease. *N Engl J Med* 2001; **344**: 1117–24.

87. DeFreyter PJ, Serruys PW. Percutaneous coronary intervention: a rapidly evolving field. *Cardiologie* 2000; **7**: 52–7.

88. Arora RR, Chou TM, Jain D *et al.* The Multicenter Study of Enhanced External Counterpulsation (MUST-EECP): effect of EECP on exercise-induced myocardial ischemia and angina episodes. *J Am Coll Cardiol* 1999; **33**: 1833–40.

89. Mannheimer C, Eliasson T, Augustinsson L-E. Electrical stimulation vs coronary artery bypass surgery in severe angina pectoris. The ESBY Study. *Circulation* 1998; **97**: 1157–63.

90. Claes G, Drott C, Wettervik C *et al.* Angina pectoris treated by thoraco-scopic sympathectomy. *Cardiovasc Surg* 1996; **4**: 830–1.

91. Khogali SS, Miller M, Rajesh PB *et al.* Video-assisted thoracoscopic sympathectomy for severe intractable angina. *Eur J Cardiovasc Surg* 1999; **Supplement 1**: S95–8.

92. Burkhoff D, Schmidt S, Schulman SP *et al.* Transmyocardial laser revascularisation compared with continued medical therapy for treat-ment of refractory angina pectoris: a prospective randomised trial. *Lancet* 1999; **354**: 885–90.

93. Aaberge L, Nordstrand K, Dragsund M *et al.* Transmyocardial revascu-larization with CO_2 laser in patients with refractory angina pectoris. Clinical results from the Norwegian Randomised Trial. *J Am Coll Cardiol* 2000; **35**: 1170–7.

94. Oesterle S, Sanborn T, Ali N *et al.* Percutaneous transmyocardial laser revascularisation for severe angina: the PACIFIC randomised trial. Potential Class Improvement From Intramyocardial Channels. *Lancet* 2000; **356**: 1705–10.

Management of unstable angina

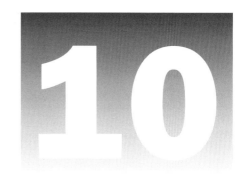

J. Brendan Foley

Introduction

Chest pain is one of the commonest medical conditions to be assessed in emergency medicine. In the USA, five million patients present to the emergency room per annum for the assessment of chest pain, with 1.7 million being admitted with suspected acute cardiac syndromes. These include acute myocardial infarction, unstable angina and non-ST-segment-elevation myocardial infarction.[1,2] The frequency of unstable angina exceeds that of acute myocardial infarction by the order of about 2:1, and this has significant resource implications. The accurate diagnosis and optimum management of unstable angina are crucial to patient welfare. Patients with unstable angina are at significant risk of myocardial infarction, with all of its potential associated complications.

The clinical syndrome of unstable angina represents an acute ischaemic threat to the heart, the definition of which has progressively evolved as the underlying pathophysiology has been clarified. Unstable angina has been known by a number of different names, including crescendo angina, pre-infarction syndrome, acute coronary insufficiency and intermediate coronary syndrome. The clinical features of unstable angina have long been recognized. They include recent-onset angina, angina at rest and progression of the symptoms of stable angina. A more structured approach was proposed in 1989, and is generally referred to as the Braunwald classification (Chapter 1, Table 1.2, p. 2). According to this classification, the degree of unstable angina is categorized on the basis of the clinical history, accelerated exertional angina or rest pain. The latter is timed with respect to presentation and the circumstances precipitating the angina. Also factored into the assessment is the presence or absence of electrocardiogram (ECG) changes and the intensity of anti-ischaemic therapy at the time of the event. This classification has been widely used in clinical trials, and has been shown to be useful for risk-stratifying

Figure 10.1
Prognostic value of troponins (TNI, troponin I; TNT, troponin T) in acute coronary syndromes. Reproduced with permission from Ham CW, Braunwald E. *Circulation* 2000; **102**: 118–22.

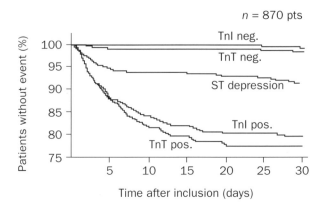

patients with unstable angina. A modification to the classification has been proposed as a result of the identification of the role of cardiac-specific troponins, which are themselves independent predictors of outcome in patients with unstable angina (see Figure 10.1).

Pathophysiology of unstable angina

Unstable angina occurs when there is an acute critical reduction in myocardial perfusion. In the majority of cases this is due to severe stenosis or occlusion in a major epicardial vessel. However, in occasional circumstances it may be aggravated by anaemia or situations of increased metabolic demand, such as severe sepsis or thyrotoxicosis. It may also be provoked or precipitated by increased wall stress, such as occurs in aortic stenosis or uncontrolled severe hypertension. The critical pathophysiological mechanisms underlying unstable angina are similar to those of acute myocardial infarction.

Ischaemic heart disease may be viewed as a clinical spectrum, with stable angina of varying degrees at one end, progressing to unstable angina, and then on to non-ST-segment elevation myocardial infarction and finally acute myocardial infarction. In the majority of cases, unstable angina is due to compromise of the myocardial blood flow caused by disruption of the atherosclerotic plaque and associated thrombus formation. There is also a degree of associated coronary vasospasm. This a dynamic feature that produces changes in blood flow in an already severely compromised situation. In its most severe form, coronary spasm may occur in the setting of an angiographically normal coronary artery, and may be of sufficient magnitude to result in acute myocardial infarction.

Plaque rupture occurs as a result of the combination of shear forces and the secretion of proteolytic enzymes by macrophages that weaken the fibrous cap and allow the continuity and integrity of the endothelium to be broken (see

Chapter 3, p. 25). Shear forces occur at branch points and regions of coronary stenosis. There is associated non-laminar flow of blood, which permits potential macrophage and neutrophil adhesion with subsequent trans-endothelial neutrophil migration. This process results in the release of proteolytic enzymes and chemotactant factors that further destabilize the plaque and accelerate the unstable process. Plaque rupture occurs in the thinned endothelium overlying the lipid core of the atherosclerotic vessel (see Plate 3.1). Plaque disruption results in exposure of the contents of the plaque to the bloodstream. This results in the adherence of platelets to the sub-endothelial matrix, with release of thromboxane A_2 and the generation of thrombin, which further amplifies the process of thrombus formation.

The importance of the lipid core (see Plate 10.1) in the pathogenesis of acute ischaemic syndromes is highlighted by observations from the trials of lipid reduction. In these trials, the reduction in the acute myocardial ischaemic events of unstable angina and myocardial infarction far outweighed that which would have been expected from the documented angiographic regression or reduction in progression. It has been proposed that this was due to plaque stabilization secondary to a reduction in the lipid core, which paralleled the reduction in serum cholesterol in the intervention groups. It has been further proposed that a key part of the progression of the atherosclerotic process is due to repeated plaque rupture, destabilization and healing. This is associated with remodelling of the vessel and ultimately an incremental reduction in the lumen. Plaque erosion is another potential mechanism involved in unstable angina. In this scenario, thrombus adheres directly to the surface of the plaque without involvement of the deeper layers of the plaque, such as the lipid core (as occurs in plaque rupture). The platelet-rich thrombus, as well as being a promoter of further platelet activation, also releases vasoconstrictor substances such as serotonin and thromboxane A_2. The importance of thrombus formation in acute ischaemic syndromes is highlighted by the key role of thrombolytic agents in the management of acute myocardial infarction and glycoprotein IIb–IIIa inhibitors in unstable angina, non-ST-segment myocardial infarctions and acute myocardial infarction. Restabilization of plaque following an episode of instability may take from weeks to months, and patients who present with unstable angina or non-ST-segment acute myocardial infarction are at increased risk of major cardiac events during the first few months, with further events occurring in 20–30% of cases.

The process of plaque destabilization with the formation of adherent thrombus is a dynamic one, the clinical outcome of which is dependent on the degree of luminal narrowing that occurs as a result of the process, and the ability of the myocardium to respond to the reduction in coronary perfusion. The clinical scenario that develops is a consequence of a heterogeneous group of variables (see Box 10.1). These include the extent and site of myocardium at risk. Clinical presentations that involve large amounts of territory and those

> **Box 10.1   Factors that affect the clinical presentation of infarction**
>
> - Infarct size
> - Anterior territory
> - Papillary muscle involvement
> - Ischaemic preconditioning
> - Hibernation
> - Collaterals

that predominantly affect the anterior circulation of the heart pose the greatest threat. Smaller key territories, such as those that may impact directly on the papillary muscles, may have greater clinical consequences than would otherwise be warranted by the amount of tissue involved. Critical ischaemia of a papillary muscle may result in severe pulmonary oedema despite the fact that only a small amount of myocardium is jeopardized. Myocardial hibernation and preconditioning are other important variables. Myocardial hibernation occurs as a consequence of chronic hypoperfusion due to a high-grade coronary stenosis. In this situation the myocardium adapts to the low flow, and complete occlusion of the vessel may not result in an acute ischaemic syndrome. In preconditioning, repeated brief episodes of myocardial hypoperfusion prepare the myocardium for a more prolonged episode of myocardial ischaemia. This process has even been seen to occur during coronary angioplasty, whereby with successive balloon inflations there may be less ST-segment change and less pain experienced by the patient. The presence of coronary collaterals is another important variable. Collaterals may be visible at coronary angiography, to occluded and critically stenosed vessels. Or they may not be visible on angiography, but may come into play in situations of greater myocardial ischaemia (this process is known as collateral recruitment).

Focal areas of myocardial necrosis have been observed in the region subserved by a vessel with an unstable plaque, and these may represent repeated episodes of thrombus embolization. These areas of focal necrosis may not be sufficient to produce a detectable rise in creatine phosphate kinase (CPK) or CPK-MB, but may result in the release of cardiac troponin I or T.

Clinical assessment

The assessment and management of the patient with possible unstable angina begin as soon as the patient is seen, and include the basic but important features of a detailed history and a general medical examination, augmented by basic investigations including ECG, chest X-ray and baseline bloods. More advanced investigations, including further blood work, exercise stress testing with or without an associated imaging modality (either nuclear scintigraphy or echocardiography), and cardiac catheterization help to further confirm or reject the diagnosis, and aid the decision-making process with regard to patient management.

Clinical presentation

The typical presentation of unstable angina is well recognized and falls into a few well-defined patterns. These include destabilization of previously stable angina such that some or all of the following features occur: episodes occurring more frequently, more easily induced, of greater intensity, lasting longer or more difficult to stabilize. New-onset angina is considered to be unstable, but especially so if it is occurring on minimum exertion or at rest, and particularly if the episodes are lasting for longer than 20 min. The setting in which rest pain occurs should also be clarified further. Emotional and intellectual stress has been shown to promote myocardial ischaemia. Angina pain is more likely to occur in the morning and also postprandially. Angina resulting in waking from sleep may be precipitated by dreams, which may be less ominous than angina waking the patient from sleep in the absence of any identifiable stimulus. The majority of patients who present with unstable angina do so with prolonged pain, with only about 20% of cases presenting with recent onset or progression of previously stable angina.

Atypical presentations may occur, and are more likely to be found in women, diabetics and the elderly. These cases may present with atypical pain, which may have gastrointestinal features including an indigestion type of sensation or epigastric pain. They may also present with stabbing chest pain or have a pleuritic component.

Chest pain is the final manifestation of myocardial ischaemia, and is not universal in all episodes or in all patients with myocardial ischaemia. Myocardial ischaemia initially causes abnormalities of myocardial contraction and relaxation. These are followed by changes in the ECG and then chest discomfort. Around 80% of episodes of myocardial ischaemia do not result in symptoms of angina, and they have been referred to as silent ischaemia. In some individuals, chest discomfort may not occur and acute myocardial ischaemia with or without infarction may present with the consequences of myocardial dysfunction, including shortness of breath and acute pulmonary oedema, or even as sudden arrhythmic death. Acute pulmonary oedema may occur in the setting of temporary ischaemia-induced papillary muscle dysfunction, which may result in reversible severe mitral incompetence, the features of which may resolve quickly with treatment – to such an extent that no murmur may be audible once the acute event has been stabilized. The history should include not only a detailed assessment of the chest discomfort but also any risk factors. The traditional risk factors, including sex, age, family history, history of hypertension, diabetes and smoking history should all be taken into account. Women tend to be protected from ischaemic heart disease during their reproductive years, and generally tend to develop myocardial ischaemic problems 10 years later than men.

The physical examination is usually unremarkable. Specific cardiac features, such as the development of an extra heart sound in the form of an S3 or S4, may occur. Other indirect features that may support an underlying vasculo-pathic type of process, such as carotid or other vascular bruits or features of peripheral vascular disease, may also be found. Clinical features that suggest an increased predisposition to vascular disease, such as arcus cornealis or xanthomata or hypertension, are also useful. In rare circumstances, features that may support an arteritis may be identified (e.g. in patients with systemic lupus erythematosus or polymyositis). Other unusual scenarios include coronary embolus in patients with prosthetic valves, especially if they are not therapeutically anticoagulated.

Electrocardiogram

It is important to emphasize that patients with unstable angina may show no abnormal ECG changes. Having said that, the resting ECG is a crucial part of the assessment of a patient presenting with possible unstable angina. Transient ECG abnormalities may be present if an ECG is performed while the patient is symptomatic, and these abnormalities may be all the more apparent when compared with an ECG when the symptoms have settled. If previous ECGs are available, new changes may be appreciated. The availability of previous ECGs is particularly useful if the patient has had a prior myocardial infarction, has left ventricular hypertrophy or presents with left bundle branch block. The presence of changes from previously documented features, even if the previous ECG was abnormal, is of prime importance in the assessment of the patient. The presence of pathological Q-waves in two or more contiguous leads provides evidence of previous myocardial infarction, which in some cases may have been silent. They constitute evidence in support of the presence of coronary artery disease, but they do not confirm that the present episode represents unstable angina. The most reliable ECG indicators of unstable angina are ST-segment changes and T-wave changes (see Chapter 8, p. 101). ST-segment depression of >1 mm in two or more contiguous leads is highly suggestive of unstable angina. Deep symmetrical T-wave inversion, especially when seen in the anterior praecordial leads, is again highly suggestive of unstable angina. ST-segment elevation in two or more contiguous leads supports a diagnosis of acute myocardial infarction, but transient ST-segment elevation may be seen in unstable angina. This is generally thought to be due to coronary vasospasm, especially in the presence of a critical coronary stenosis producing intermittent coronary occlusion. Occasionally, coronary spasm may occur in the setting of an angiographically normal coronary artery, resulting in ST-segment elevation. This has traditionally been referred to as Prinzmetal's angina. As noted previously, only about 20% of episodes of myocardial ischaemia result in chest discomfort. Continuous ST-segment monitoring may detect episodes of ST-segment change indicative of myocardial ischaemia without the occurrence of chest pain. Continuous ST-segment monitoring is often employed in the initial evaluation of patients with chest pain syndromes, and may not only be useful for identifying the presence of ischaemic heart disease and thus establishing a diagnosis, but may also be used to monitor the response of the patient to treatment. Thus it aids the identification of those who are responding to the medical therapy that has been instituted, and it also helps to identify those who require more aggressive management.

Chest X-ray

A standard postero-anterior and lateral chest X-ray is a useful screening test for excluding significant pulmonary lesions, providing information on heart size and potentially suggesting aortic dissection. However, if aortic dissection is considered to have real potential in the differential diagnosis, more focused tests in that regard, such as transthoracic and transoesophageal echocardiography, spiral CT scan, aortogram or magnetic resonance imaging, need to be performed as a matter of urgency.

Biochemical markers

The traditional markers of myocardial ischaemia have been creatine kinase (CK) and its cardiac isoenzyme (CK-MB). These are markers of myocardial necrosis. They have been superseded by the cardiac troponins, which are now the recommended markers of myocardial necrosis. The troponins are released from cardiac myocytes after even minor amounts of myocardial cell loss. The troponins are structural proteins located in the thin filaments of the contractile apparatus of cardiac and skeletal muscle. There are three distinct structural proteins (troponins I, C and T), and commercial kits are available for the measurement of troponins I and T. Troponins regulate the calcium-dependent interaction of myosin and actin. The cardiac isoforms are encoded in specific genes and can be differentiated by monoclonal antibodies. Thus the detection of cardiac troponin I or T is specific for myocardial necrosis and, once detected, the patient is then diagnosed as having an acute myocardial infarct. In the setting of ST-segment-elevation acute myocardial infarction, there is a rise in troponin levels within 3–4 h, and they remain elevated for many days. Their rate of appearance and clearance in non-ST-segment-elevation myocardial infarction is less well defined, but they generally rise within 12 h and remain elevated for up to 14 days. The initial rise is due to troponin release from the cytoplasmic pool, and the continued release is due to proteolysis of contractile proteins which may last for up to 2 weeks.

Samples need to be drawn for up to 12 h after presentation, and repeated sampling is necessary. As a result of this prolonged elevation, troponins are not useful for the detection of repeat myocardial infarction during the first 2 weeks, and repeat elevation of CK is more useful for determining whether repeated infarction has occurred. Measurement of the other cardiac enzymes, including the widely used CK with its MB isoform, will continue to be useful because of this and also due to their widespread availability and relatively low cost. It has been noted that elevation of troponin levels may occur in renal failure and pulmonary embolus. It has been proposed that this may represent a false elevation, or alternatively that it may be due to minute amounts of myocardial cell death caused by myocardial stretch in the setting of large pulmonary emboli and silent infarcts in patients with renal failure (a population with a high frequency of advanced cardiac disease).

Other biochemical parameters that impact on the patient risk factor profile, such as elevated cholesterol and blood glucose levels, are of importance. Not only do they identify an adverse risk factor profile for the patient, but they are amenable to modulation with appropriate dietary advice, weight reduction (if necessary) and medication. A full blood count will occasionally reveal features that may aggravate angina. These include significant anaemia or conditions that may increase the potential for thrombosis, such as essential thrombocythaemia. Biochemical and haematological parameters that may have a role but which are not yet generally available include serum homocysteine, high-sensitivity C-reactive protein (CRP), fibrinogen level and lipoprotein(a) (Lpa). In patients in whom myocardial infarction may occur as part of a systemic inflammatory illness, other biochemical markers, such as lupus anticoagulant or antiphospholipid antibody, which are associated with an increased thrombotic tendency may need to be measured.

Stress testing

Exercise stress testing helps to establish the diagnosis of ischaemic heart disease, especially if the resting ECG is normal and if the blood work has been unremarkable. The accuracy of stress testing may be augmented by the addition of nuclear perfusion imaging or echocardiography (see Chapter 8, p. 108). These techniques may be of particular use in patients in whom the baseline ECG has abnormal features, such as left bundle branch block, left ventricular hypertrophy and strain, or features of previous myocardial infarction, or in those with a pre-excited ECG, as occurs in Wolff–Parkinson–White syndrome. It is reasonable practice to perform standard exercise stress testing without the addition of these other features, looking for the hallmark of ST-segment depression of 1 mm or more measured 80 ms after the J-point in two or more contiguous leads. ST-segment elevation of 2 mm or more in two or more contiguous leads may also occur, representing an abnormal response. Associated features are important, too, including the development of chest discomfort suggestive of the presenting angina, exercise-associated hypotension (a reduction in systolic pressure of 20 mmHg or more) or the induction of ventricular arrhythmias. An early positive stress test has been thought to identify those at increased risk of further events, but the hard-and-fast data to support this have been lacking. The standard protocol used is that of Bruce, and it has been demonstrated to be safe to perform in patients presenting with unstable angina 24 h after the last episode of chest pain, assuming that the patient is fully ambulant and does not have any other adverse features, such as heart failure or uncontrolled significant hypertension. More recently, stress testing has been performed within 8 h of resolution of chest pain in selected patients who are haemodynamically stable and in whom troponins and serial ECGs have not shown any features of myocardial necrosis.

Echocardiography

Echocardiography is useful in that it provides details of the parameter of left ventricular function, which is an important independent variable in stratifying patient risk. Echocardiography may also identify regions of segmental wall abnormalities, which would support the diagnosis of myocardial infarction. An echocardiogram that is performed during an episode of chest pain may reveal a segment of decreased wall movement that may recover following resolution of the pain. Again this would support an ischaemic aetiology of the pain. Stress echocardiography involves the administration of an agent that increases myocardial workload (see Chapter 8, p. 110). A negative stress echocardiogram is associated with a very low serious 1-year event rate.

Cardiac catheterization

Cardiac catheterization and coronary angiography provide unique information about the presence or absence of angiographic disease, and help to identify the extent of coronary stenoses and the myocardium at risk. Coronary angiograms provide images of the inner lumen of the coronary artery, but do

Figure 10.2
Right coronary artery with extensive disease, collaterals and acute distal occlusion.

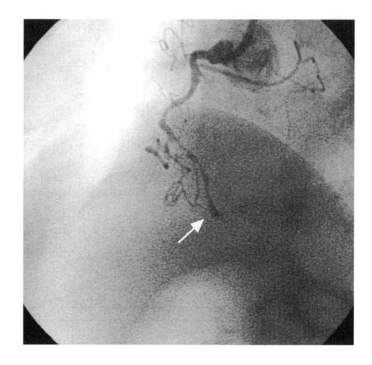

not provide information about the lumen itself. It is recognized that remodelling of the coronary artery occurs, whereby the initial effect of atheromatous disease in the coronary artery is to cause expansion of the coronary artery without reduction of the lumen. As the process continues, this is followed by a progressive reduction in the diameter of the coronary lumen and compromise of myocardial blood flow with its associated consequences (see Figure 10.2). Features of intracoronary thrombus are identified at coronary angiography in about 20% of patients with unstable angina. These include overhanging edges suggestive of ulceration, irregularity, a filling defect surrounded by contrast, or occlusion of the vessel without tapering. Angioscopic studies have identified thrombus in 60–70% of patients.

A diffuse process may occur within the coronary vasculature that results in a uniform deposition of atheroma throughout the coronary vessels. As there may be no focal stenosis or even edge irregularity, the angiogram may appear normal. In the short to medium term the prognosis is good, but disease progression may occur over a period of years with the development of focal stenosis. Newer imaging modalities, including intravascular ultrasound, may identify this process but are not suitable for the routine assessment of coronary artery disease. One situation where intravascular ultrasound has been used is in the surveillance of the accelerated atherosclerosis that tends to occur following cardiac transplantation. Magnetic resonance imaging has yielded some spectacular images of coronary arteries, providing details not

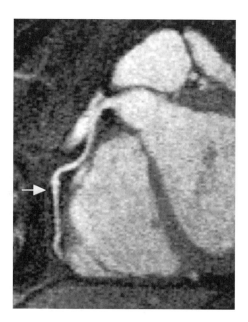

Figure 10.3
Magnetic resonance angiogram (MRA) with normal right coronary artery. (Courtesy Dr J. Meaney.)

only of the lumen but also of the wall of the coronary artery (see Figure 10.3). However, as yet the results must be regarded as experimental, and they cannot be obtained reliably in all patients. Further development will be necessary before this imaging modality becomes reliable and widely available.

Management

Once a diagnosis of unstable angina has been entertained as the working diagnosis, the patient must be admitted to hospital. If there is already evidence of myocardial necrosis, as evidenced by an elevation of troponin levels or other markers of cell death, without the classic features of myocardial infarction on the ECG, the patient needs to be admitted to a monitoring facility, ideally the coronary care unit or a step-down unit. If there is no elevation of cardiac-specific enzymes, a bed with telemetry monitoring is suitable. Ideally, a multi-lead ECG facility with the ability to generate a continuous 12-lead ECG is needed, but this is not yet standard equipment, and is still undergoing clinical evaluation.

The initial consideration is to ensure that active myocardial ischaemia has passed and that for any associated features, such as pulmonary oedema or hypotension, treatment has either been given or is in hand. Indicators of continuing ischaemia include ischaemic discomfort or continuing dynamic ECG changes on monitoring. If the patient is not already on *aspirin*, they should receive an immediate dose of 75–150 mg, often administered acutely

> **Box 10.2   Drugs that are used in the management of unstable angina**
>
> - Oxygen
> - Aspirin/clopidogrel
> - Heparin/low-molecular-weight heparin (LMWH)
> - Nitrates (sublingual/intravenous)
> - Beta-blockers
> - Calcium-channel blockers
> - Glycoprotein IIb/IIIa antagonists

in a soluble form, followed by 75 mg per day (see Box 10.2). If the patient has a clear contraindication to aspirin or aspirin allergy, oral clopidogrel at 300 mg, followed by 75 mg per day may be used. *Clopidogrel* is an adenosine diphosphate receptor antagonist. The addition of clopidogrel to aspirin effects a modest reduction in nonfatal myocardial infarction, but increases the risk of bleeding (CURE).[13]

If there is evidence of ongoing myocardial ischaemia, the patient should receive sublingual nitroglycerine 200–400 mcg. If there is then continuing evidence of myocardial ischaemia, they should be treated with an intravenous infusion of nitroglycerine. Oral or topical *nitrate* preparations can be substituted and titrated upward according to the symptom status of the patient and side-effects such as headache or hypotension.

Early consideration should be given to the institution of *beta-blockers* if the patient is not already receiving them. If they are already receiving them, the dose should be assessed, aiming for a resting heart rate of 50–60 beats/min. Before initiating or increasing beta-blockers, the haemodynamic status of the patient needs to be considered with regard to evidence of heart failure or hypotension. Occasionally it is necessary to administer beta-blockers intravenously, but they are more often administered orally. An indication for rapid beta-blockade, possibly by the intravenous route, is continuing angina in the presence of a relative tachycardia without evidence of congestive cardiac failure or hypotension. Short-acting oral beta-blockers allow rapid upwards titration, with increments every 4–6 h, depending on the drug, until the desired heart rate is achieved. This may be limited by the appearance of problems such as bronchospasm, hypotension, heart failure, significant bradycardia or heart block, which may require withholding of the beta-blocker or a reduction in the dose. Once they are established on the beta-blocker, the patient can be changed to a once-daily long-acting beta-blocker that does not cross the blood–brain barrier significantly, to reduce the frequency of peripheral side-effects and improve compliance.

Calcium-channel blockers are commonly used in the setting of unstable angina, but data on their use in this setting are scarce. The data that exist suggest that they provide symptom relief in patients who are already receiving nitrates and beta-blockers. They may be of use in those with contraindications to beta-blockers and in those with Prinzmetal's variant angina. It is recommended that dihydropyridines and especially the short-acting dihydropyridines (e.g. the standard formulation of nifedipine) should not be used without the concomitant use of a beta-blocker.

Anticoagulation with *intravenous heparin* should be initiated as soon as is possible if there are no contraindications to its use. *Low-molecular-weight heparin* preparations have the advantages of providing more reliable anticoagulation, ease of subcutaneous administration and do not require monitoring to determine the degree of anticoagulation. The dose administered is determined by the weight of the patient. Care needs to be taken that the injections are truly subcutaneous, as intramuscular injections may result in severe blood loss into the anterior abdominal wall. Low-molecular-weight heparins have the disadvantage of not being readily reversed in the event of a bleeding complication – a problem in the event of emergency cardiac catheterization or cannulation of a central vein for central haemodynamic monitoring. If it is necessary to proceed to emergency percutaneous revascularization or coronary artery bypass surgery in a patient who is on a low-molecular-weight heparin, the exact degree of anticoagulation of the patient who is to undergo the procedure cannot be easily determined, and the potential dose of heparin required for the procedure is unknown. This may also impact on potential bleeding complications if a glycoprotein IIb/IIIa antagonist is necessary. The disadvantages of unfractionated heparin include its variable anticoagulant effect, resulting in the need for frequent assessments of anticoagulation. It also results in less inhibition of clot-bound thrombin than of fluid-phase thrombin, and has a greater potential to produce heparin-induced thrombocytopenia than low-molecular-weight heparins. Randomized trials of the use of either low-molecular-weight heparins or unfractionated heparin have demonstrated modest superiority of low-molecular-weight heparins. In clinical practice, the ease of use and reliability of low-molecular-weight heparins favour their use, but in patients in whom it is thought that invasive procedures may need to be performed urgently, it would be reasonable to treat them with unfractionated heparin during the period of instability. The duration of anticoagulation is usually for 24–48 h following stabilization of the patient.

Glycoprotein IIb/IIIa antagonists (see Box 10.3) have been shown to be of benefit in patients who present with unstable angina, with most benefit being seen in those in whom percutaneous revascularization procedures are performed.[3] The integrin glycoprotein IIb/IIIa receptor is located on the platelet surface membrane. It binds circulating fibrinogen and von Willebrand

---

Box 10.3   Glycoprotein IIb/IIIa inhibitors

- Abciximab (Reopro)
- Eptifibatide (Integrilin)
- Tirofiban (Aggrastat)

---

factor and cross-links platelets, and is the final common pathway in platelet aggregation. The glycoprotein IIb/IIIa antagonists block the receptor, preventing the binding of associated adhesion molecules, and are potent inhibitors of platelet aggregation. Three of these antagonists are approved for clinical use, with others currently undergoing clinical evaluation. *Abciximab* is human–murine chimeric monoclonal antibody fragment that binds with high affinity to the glycoprotein IIb/IIIa receptor, from which it has a slow dissociation rate. Abciximab is not specific for the glycoprotein IIb/IIIa receptor, and has equal affinity for the vitronectin receptor, which plays a role in cell adhesion, migration and proliferation. *Eptifibatide* (a cyclic heptapeptide) and *tirofiban* (a non-peptide mimetic) are highly specific for the glycoprotein IIb/IIIa receptor, with rapid reversible pharmokinetics and short plasma half-lives. Platelet aggregation is inhibited in a dose-dependent manner, with almost complete inhibition of thrombosis at 80% receptor occupancy. Following discontinuation of abciximab, platelet function returns to normal over a period of 12–36 h. Normalization of platelet function occurs over 30–40 min following cessation of the reversible inhibitors. When using glycoprotein IIb/IIIa inhibitors it is necessary to reduce the amount of heparin used, with lower bolus and infusions in those undergoing percutaneous revasularization procedures. In those in whom significant bleeding occurs, the glycoprotein IIb/IIIa inhibitor needs to be stopped. In the case of abciximab, a platelet infusion needs to be started after the period of 10–30 min that is necessary for the clearance of circulating drug. After transfusion of the platelets, abciximab redistributes to the transfused platelets, reducing the mean receptor blockade. Platelet transfusion is rarely necessary with eptifibatide and tirofiban, and may not be effective during the 2-h period that is required for the elimination of these agents from the circulating plasma. Serious thrombocytopenia may occur rarely (in less than 1% of patients). It is recommended that the platelet count should be checked about 4 h after the initiation of therapy with these agents, and repeated every 6–8 h during their use. Development of a human antichimeric antibody occurs in about 5% of patients following the administration of abciximab, but no instances of hypersensitivity were documented in a registry of repeat administration in 500 patients, although the frequency of thrombocytopenia was somewhat increased. No such antibody response has been observed with eptifibatide and tirofiban.

Although the role of glycoprotein IIb/IIIa inhibitors in patients with unstable angina who are undergoing percutaneous revascularization procedures is well established, their role in other patients with unstable angina has yet to be defined fully. Their use has been recommended in the American College of Cardiology/American Heart Association/European Society of Cardiology guidelines for unstable angina, but these were written before the recent GUSTO IV-ACS study[4] results became available. This was a large randomized trial of abciximab, and it did not show a significant benefit. However, the small molecules eptifibatide and tirofiban have been associated with reductions in combined 30-day death and recurrent cardiac events after admission with unstable coronary syndromes, although there was no long-term effect on mortality.[5] Their use is also limited by their cost, and their role in subgroups of patients with unstable angina needs to be defined further. It is possible that individuals with a high thrombus burden will benefit most from their use. The studies of unstable angina to date have included patients with ECG changes and in some instances abnormal cardiac enzymes. Ideally, methods of identifying patients who would derive maximum benefit from the use of these agents need to be found.

The pace of clinical investigation and the rate at which the patient moves through the various assessments that are performed depend on the clinical scenario. If the patient continues to show features of ongoing ischaemia, or if they have had significant haemodynamic compromise at presentation, such as pulmonary oedema or hypotension, they need to be considered for more aggressive management. This includes early assessment of left ventricular function by echocardiography and cardiac catheterization and coronary angiography. If the patient is not already on a glycoprotein IIb/IIIa inhibitor before being taken to the catheterization laboratory, consideration should be given to initiation of one before starting the angiogram, as in many cases percutaneous revascularization may be performed immediately. Coronary stent implantation has been shown to be safe in the setting of acute myocardial infarction, and is therefore reasonable in the setting of unstable angina. In both stable angina and acute myocardial infarction, stent implantation results in a less frequent need for subsequent target lesion revascularization than balloon angioplasty alone, and the same benefit is probably conferred in unstable angina.

In those patients who settle with conservative measures following admission, a risk factor analysis needs to be performed and modifiable risk factors addressed. Patients need to be stratified with regard to short-, intermediate- and long-term risk. The presence of a long pre-existing history of ischaemic heart disease, prior myocardial infarction and important risk factors, such as diabetes or marked hyperlipidaemia, help to identify those at increased risk of further events. Factors such as age and general health of the patient need to be considered. Although as a general rule elderly patients tend to have a worse short-term and intermediate-term risk factor profile than younger patients, each patient must be assessed individually to determine whether extensive investigation is warranted. In elderly patients and those with severe coexisting illness, a clinical decision may be made only to assess matters further if the patient continues to display ongoing symptoms of ischaemia, or if they had significant haemodynamic compromise at presentation. Invasive testing is associated with an increased risk in elderly patients, which is further elevated in the setting of unstable angina. Two novel serum markers of short-term recurrence risk have now become available, namely the cardiomyofibrillary protein troponin T (or I) and high-sensitivity CRP, and the former has become established in many clinical practices. Troponin T or I identifies patients at higher risk of recurrent ischaemia. The short-term 40-day clinical recurrence was 14% in troponin-T-positive patients with unstable angina in the recent FRISC study,[6] and 4.7% in troponin-negative patients. CRP is discussed in more detail in Chapter 3 (p. 41), but will not become clinically useful until high-sensitivity assays are routinely available.

There are reasonable data to support a conservative approach to the management of patients with unstable angina, with the most compelling data coming from the VANQWISH study,[7] in which patients who presented with unstable angina fared better with a conservative approach. However, the Tactics/TIMI 18 trial[8] recently studied unstable angina patients receiving the glycoprotein IIb/IIIa antagonist tirofiban. In those patients who were randomized to early invasive therapy (i.e. automatic early angiography with appropriate revascularization), the primary end-point of death, myocardial infarction and recurrent acute coronary syndromes at 6 months was reduced from 19.4% to 15.9% by an aggressive approach, with an even greater benefit in tropinin-T-positive patients.

In those patients in whom a conservative approach is being considered as the first option, an assessment of left ventricular function with echocardiography is necessary to identify individuals with significant impairment of left ventricular function, so that they can be treated with angiotensin-converting-enzyme inhibitors and beta-blockers.

The presence of recurrent chest pain, early positive exercise tests and positive nuclear scintigraphy or stress echocardiography tests all help to identify patients who require early coronary angiography. Inducible reversible ischaemia on isotope perfusion scanning or stress echocardiography, especially if there is a large amount of myocardium at risk, is also an indication for coronary angiography.

Angiography in unstable angina

The general risks associated with a cardiac catheterization and coronary angiography in the setting of unstable angina are slightly higher than in stable angina. Other features associated with increased risk at angiography include advanced age, impaired renal function, diabetes mellitus, diffuse arterial disease (including peripheral vascular disease) and carotid disease. Recent myocardial infarction is also a risk, and there is a risk of embolic events from left ventricular thrombus that may occur following acute myocardial infarction. Commonly, echocardiography is performed before the angiogram in order to exclude the presence of left ventricular thrombus, and the left ventricular angiogram may be omitted from the assessment at angiography. The risk of coronary angiography in the setting of unstable angina or recent myocardial infarction is generally 1% or less of procedure-related myocardial infarction, 0.001% of stroke or death and 1% of significant access site complications. Commonly, percutaneous revascularization may be performed at the same time if suitable anatomy is identified. The risks of percutaneous revascularization are slightly higher than in stable angina, but would generally be associated with a 4–12% risk of myocardial infarction, depending on the definition of myocardial infarction used, and would be lower if a glycoprotein IIb/IIIa inhibitor was given at the time of the intervention.

Adjunctive devices are available and under development for specific subsets of patients with specific morphological or anatomical challenges to revascularization. These include the following:

- *rotational atherectomy devices* which drill calcified lesions using a 10-μ-diameter diamond drill to reduce debris to < 10 μ, thus allowing capillary washout;
- *directional coronary atherectomy devices* which core away bulky eccentric plaques with an apple-core-like device;
- *laser atherectomy* which cuts and debulks tissue using an argon laser;
- *suction/extraction devices* to clear degenerated saphenous vein grafts prior to angioplasty;
- *drug-coated and radiation-coated stents* which have the exciting potential to reduce rates of restenosis (the principal limitation of coronary stenting).

The indications for revascularization depend on the status of the patient, the presence and extent of ischaemia induced at stress testing, and the extent of disease identified at coronary angiography. A number of anatomical subtypes have been identified that are associated with a better survival with surgical intervention. These include significant left main stem disease, significant three-vessel disease (especially if associated with impaired left ventricular function) and two-vessel disease (associated with proximal left anterior descending coronary disease). The studies (BARI and CASS)[9,10] date from the early 1980s and pre-date many of the practices that are now considered to be standard care, including the widespread use of aspirin, beta-blockers, angiotensin-converting-enzyme inhibitors and lipid-lowering agents. These studies compared surgical intervention with medical therapy, and also pre-dated the widespread use of percutaneous revasularization procedures. A number of studies have compared angioplasty and stenting with coronary bypass, and have shown equivalency with regard to safety, but better freedom from angina for surgery and a greater need for repeat interventions in the first year in the angioplasty and stent groups (ARTS).[11] The recurrence of angina and the need for repeat procedures are most often due to renarrowing of the dilated segment (a process known as restenosis). This has been reduced by the widespread use of stents, but when in-stent restenosis occurs it can be associated with an aggressive process with a high potential for recurrence. There are data to support a better long-term outcome in diabetics with multi-vessel disease treated with coronary artery bypass surgery. Newer, exciting technologies involving the development of stents that deliver drugs which combat the potential for restenosis hold promise and may reduce the need for repeat interventions (RAVEL).[12] This is an ever-changing area, and yesterdays' orthodoxies are constantly being outdated.

Summary

Unstable angina presents a serious diagnostic and therapeutic challenge to the admitting physician. Antiplatelet and antithrombotic therapy should be instituted immediately, the patient should be risk-stratified rapidly, and nitrates, beta-blockers and lipid-lowering therapy should be instituted where appropriate. There is still controversy over whether patients should undergo early angiography or be investigated on an ischaemia-driven basis. There are conflicting data on the importance of glycoprotein IIb/IIIa inhibitors in acute coronary syndrome in the absence of a plan for revascularization, and further studies are awaited. Acute coronary syndrome has a high short-term recurrence rate and a significant mortality. Its incidence has overtaken that of myocardial infarction, and it will impact on hospital practice for many years to come.

References

1. Hlatky MA. Evaluation of chest pain in the emergency department. *N Engl J Med* 1997; **337**: 1687–9.
2. Mehta RH, Eagle KA. Missed diagnoses of acute coronary syndromes in the emergency room – continuing challenges. *N Engl J Med* 2000; **342**: 1207–10.
3. EPILOG investigators. Platelet glycoprotein IIb/IIIa receptor blockade and low-dose heparin during percutaneous coronary revascularization. *N Engl J Med* 1997; **336**: 1689–96.

4. GUSTO IV-ACS investigators. Effect of glycoprotein IIb/IIIa receptor blocker abciximab on outcome in patients with acute coronary syndromes without early coronary revascularisation. *Lancet* 2001; **357**: 1915–24.

5. Kong DF, Califf RM, Miller DP *et al.* Clinical outcomes of therapeutic agents that block the platelet gpIIb/IIIA integrin in ischaemic heart disease. *Circulation* 1998; **98**: 2829–35.

6. Lindahl B, Venge P, Wallentin L *et al.* Troponin T identifies patients with unstable coronary disease who benefit from long-term antithrombotic protection. *J Am Coll Cardiol* 1997; **29**: 43–8.

7. Boden WE, O'Rourke RA, Cawford MH *et al.* Outcomes in patients with acute non-Q-wave myocardial infarction randomly assigned to an invasive as compared with a conservative management strategy. *N Engl J Med* 1998; **338**: 1785–92.

8. Cannon CP, Weinbruss WS, Dermapoulos LA *et al.* Comparison of early invasive and conservative strategies in patients with unstable coronary syndromes treated with tirofiban. *N Engl J Med* 2001; **344**: 1879–87.

9. BARI investigators. Comparison of coronary bypass surgery with angioplasty in patients with multivessel disease. *N Engl J Med* 1996; **335**: 217–25.

10. Hamm CW, Reimers J, Ischinger T *et al.* A randomized study of coronary angioplasty compared with bypass surgery in patients with symptomatic multivessel coronary disease. *N Engl J Med* 1994; **331**: 1037–43.

11. Serruys PW, Unger F, Sousa JE *et al.* Comparison of coronary bypass surgery with angioplasty in patients with multivessel disease. *N Engl J Med* 2001; **344**: 1117–24.

12. Morice M-C, Serruys PW, Sousa JE *et al.* A randomized comparsion of a sirolimus-eluting stent with a standard stent for coronary revascularization. *N Engl J Med* 2002; **346**; 1773–80.

13. Yusuf S, Zhao F, Mehta SR *et al.* Effect of clopidogrel in addition to aspirin in patients with acute coronary syndromes without ST-segment elevation. *N Engl J Med* 2001; **345(7)**: 495–502.

Surgery for angina

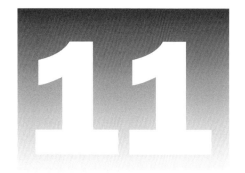

Eilis McGovern

Introduction

Myocardial revascularization is the most common surgical procedure performed in the Western world today. Over 25 000 cases of this procedure were carried out in the UK in 2000. It was known for decades that angina was due to myocardial ischaemia, and in the 1950s Vineberg performed an operation in which the internal mammary artery was implanted directly into the left ventricular myocardium in an effort to improve the blood supply to the heart.[1] However, it was not until the advent of coronary arteriography (which allowed the coronary anatomy to be outlined) and cardiopulmonary bypass (to support the circulation during heart surgery) that direct coronary artery anastomoses could be fashioned.

Favaloro performed the first coronary artery bypass operations in the 1960s and 1970s. Improvements in anaesthesia and myocardial protection resulted in an explosion in the number of operations being performed. In the 1980s, analysis of the large controlled trials comparing coronary artery surgery with medical therapy alone resulted in better patient selection, and the demonstrated long-term benefit of the internal mammary artery graft to the left anterior descending artery (LAD) resulted in its widespread use.[2]

In the 1990s, the use of thrombolysis and interventional cardiology techniques altered the referral patterns for cardiac surgery. The concept of arterial revascularization and the emergence of minimally invasive surgical techniques, in terms of both smaller incisions and off-pump surgery, have changed clinical practice, especially during the last 5 years. The new millennium is seeing a completely different patient population being referred for coronary artery surgery. The patients are older, have more advanced disease and more comorbidity, and there are more female patients. Instead of a single uniform operation being performed, the operation is now tailored to meet the needs of the individual patient, with variation in the incision, the use of the heart–lung machine, and conduit selection. Despite the changing population of patients, the overall results of coronary artery surgery are excellent, with low mortality and morbidity rates, even in high-risk groups.[3]

Patient selection

There are two main objectives of surgery in the management of patients with angina, first to improve quality of life by relieving angina symptoms, and second to improve life expectancy. In many patients both of these objectives will be achieved.

Patient selection for surgery is dependent on symptom status and the extent of coronary disease as demonstrated at coronary angiography. The effectiveness of medical therapy and the suitability of the case for angioplasty and stenting also influence the type of patient now coming forward for surgery and the surgical options available. Improved education now means that patients have more input into the process, and this has a major bearing on procedure choice in some health-care systems.

Surgery for symptoms

Patients with troublesome angina that is unresponsive to medical therapy should be offered coronary bypass surgery if they are unsuitable for interventional cardiology techniques. This is especially relevant to patients with unstable angina, where the risk of myocardial infarction and death can be significantly reduced.

Surgery for life expectancy

Several major trials conducted in the 1970s to compare medical therapy with surgical treatment for symptomatic patients with coronary artery disease demonstrated improved long-term survival in several subgroups. Trials and registries, which included the Coronary Artery Surgery Study (CASS)[4] and the European Coronary Surgery Study (ECSS),[5] showed a significant benefit of surgery over medical therapy in terms of symptom control, and in certain subgroups a definite prognostic benefit. Although some of these trials are in many ways out of date, their results still strongly influence patient selection for surgery today. Suitable patients include those with significant anatomical obstruction resulting in large areas of jeopardized myocardium, regardless of their symptoms. They include patients with:

- left mainstem disease greater than 50%;
- triple-vessel coronary disease and two-vessel disease where one of the lesions involves the proximal LAD.

Life expectancy appears to be particularly enhanced in the presence of poor left ventricular function. Thus, paradoxically, those patients with the highest surgical risk have the most to gain. In practice there is a large overlap between these two groups of patients (i.e. those being operated on for symptomatic reasons and those being operated on to improve life expectancy). Most of the patients undergoing coronary artery surgery in the current era straddle both groups and therefore benefit in two ways. However, it is important to distinguish between these two groups of patients, both to aid patient selection and to inform patients accurately about the expectations with regard to benefits from surgery.

Most patients today with single-vessel or two-vessel coronary disease would be treated by interventional cardiology techniques as a matter of choice.[6,7] Patients who are referred for surgery with this type of anatomical disease have often undergone a previous attempt at angioplasty which was technically unsuccessful, or they perhaps had lesions which were unsuitable for angioplasty (e.g. lengthy occlusions). Recurrent restenosis following angioplasty/stenting is also an indication for surgery in these circumstances.

Contraindications to coronary artery bypass surgery

The long-term success of coronary bypass surgery is related to prolonged graft patency ensuring freedom from angina.

- Patients with small and diseased coronary vessels (e.g. as seen in diabetics) are sometimes unsuitable for surgery because graft patency in these circumstances is poor.
- Patients with very poor ventricular function and congestive cardiac failure, especially where the failure symptoms are dominant, are generally unsuitable for surgery. However, if there is evidence of reversible ischaemia or if there is a localized ventricular aneurysm that is suitable for resection, surgery can be performed with good success rates.
- Patients with an established acute myocardial infarction of duration more than 6 h are unsuitable for surgery, as are patients after prolonged cardiac arrest.

Preoperative preparation

The preoperative preparation of cardiac surgical patients is best undertaken in a designated pre-admission clinic. Routine tests include chest X-ray, electrocardiogram (ECG), full blood count, renal and liver profile, coagulation screen, and group and cross-match. Attention is paid to the conduits which may be used during surgery (e.g. the presence of varicose veins in the legs, and an Allen's test for suitability of the radial artery).

Peripheral pulses are assessed, with particular attention being paid to the carotid arteries. Elderly patients, patients with diffuse peripheral vascular disease, those with a past history of a transient ischaemic attack (TIA) or stroke and those with carotid bruits should have carotid Doppler studies performed.

Patients with known chronic obstructive pulmonary disease should have pulmonary function tests performed to provide baseline data. Smokers should be encouraged to give up their habit, not just for long-term secondary prevention of coronary disease, but also to reduce the risk of postoperative respiratory complications.

Surgical technique

The standard coronary artery bypass operation is performed through a median sternotomy. The conduits are harvested first (e.g. the long saphenous vein from the leg, the radial artery or the internal mammary artery). Cardiopulmonary bypass is instituted using mild hypothermia and the

Figure 11.1
Sternotomy incision and visualization of LAD artery (arrow) on anterior surface of the heart (courtesy of Miss M. Jahangiri).

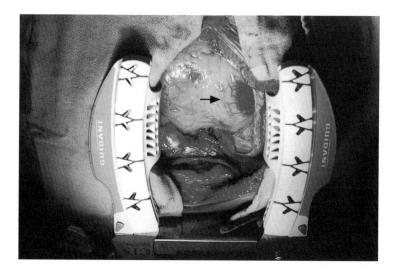

preferred method of myocardial preservation. The coronary vessels are inspected and sites for grafting are chosen in relation to angiographic findings (see Figure 11.1). Most commonly the distal anastomoses are performed first, followed by the proximal anastomoses. Cardiopulmonary bypass is discontinued and the grafts are assessed for satisfactory function. Some surgical units measure and record graft flow using Doppler probes.

Fast-tracking is a term used to describe rapid extubation following cardiac surgery, associated with short intensive-care stays and a shorter hospital stay. Most coronary artery bypass cases can be fast-tracked, and discharged on postoperative day 5 or 6.

Choice of conduit

This is individualized for each patient. The most common combination of conduits used would be the left internal mammary artery to the LAD and the saphenous vein to the other coronary vessels. The use of the left internal mammary artery in this setting has been shown to result in improved life expectancy and longer angina-free intervals.[2] In older patients, quality of life in the short term takes priority over enhanced life expectancy, and in very elderly patients many surgeons would use vein grafts alone. However, in very young patients, life expectancy assumes major importance, and there is a trend towards the use of more arterial grafts in an effort to prolong the effectiveness of the operation. Ten years after coronary artery bypass grafting, 90–95% of left internal mammary arteries have been found to be patent, whereas up to 75% of vein grafts may be occluded or severely diseased.[8] It is not uncommon to use both mammary arteries[9,10] in combination with other arterial grafts (e.g. the radial artery and, rarely, the gastro-epiploic artery or the inferior epigastric artery) in these circumstances. Recent meta-analyses suggest that a survival benefit is obtained by using two internal mammary arteries rather than one, with improved patency rates.[11] In diabetic patients, the use of bilateral internal mammary artery grafts is not recommended because of the higher incidence of sternal wound complications. The internal mammary artery is also unsuitable for use in patients who have had previous radiotherapy to the mediastinum.

Coronary endarterectomy

Occasionally, in patients who have diffuse disease and poor distal vessels, it is necessary to perform a coronary endarterectomy prior to placing the distal anastomosis. The patency of bypass grafts used in this setting is poor.

Associated procedures

Other complications of coronary artery disease, and other coincidental valve/aortic root lesions, may need to be addressed at the same time as coronary artery bypass surgery. For example:

- left ventricular aneurysmectomy;
- mitral valve repair related to papillary muscle dysfunction following myocardial infarction or annular dilatation related to congestive cardiac failure;
- aortic valve replacement for concomitant aortic stenosis.

Results

The overall mortality rate for coronary artery bypass surgery is 2–3%.[3] For many low-risk individuals undergoing elective surgery, this risk is as low as 1% or less. Higher mortality risks are associated with increasing age, female gender, poor left ventricular function, reoperation and associated diseases. It is possible to calculate the risk by using risk stratification scores such as the Parsonnet score or the Euroscore.

Morbidity following coronary artery surgery can affect any organ in the body, due to the nature of the cardiopulmonary bypass.

- *Excess bleeding* is common due to various factors, such as the coagulopathy associated with cardiopulmonary bypass and the preoperative use of agents such as heparin, aspirin and clopidogrel. Reoperative surgery is also associated with a higher risk of bleeding. In a small percentage of patients, a return to the operating theatre is required for control of bleeding.
- *Stroke* is an uncommon but devastating complication of cardiac surgery, occurring in approximately 2–3% of patients overall. It is more commonly seen in the elderly, in patients with peripheral vascular disease and in those with a previous history of stroke or TIA. High-risk patients should have carotid Doppler studies performed prior to surgery. It is thought that many perioperative neurological events are related to embolism of aortic atheromatous plaque which is mobilized during surgery. Neurological damage can also result from hypoperfusion in patients with severe pre-existing carotid stenosis, although there is controversy over the real incidence of subtle neurological impairment.[12]
- *Renal dysfunction* is uncommon in patients with normal preoperative renal indices. However, patients with pre-existing chronic renal dysfunction often experience a deterioration in their condition, resulting in a requirement for dialysis in a small number of cases.

- *Arrhythmias* are very common following cardiac surgery. Supraventricular arrhythmias, especially atrial fibrillation, occur in up to 30% of patients. They are more likely to occur in the elderly, and following the withdrawal of preoperative beta-blockers. Several studies have shown that either beta-blockers or amiodarone may decrease the postoperative incidence of atrial fibrillation.[13]

Coronary artery surgery is regarded as clean surgery, and therefore wound infection rates are low. Problems are more commonly seen in the leg wounds, especially if vein has been harvested from the groin region.

Long-term results

The more extensive the coronary artery disease, especially in the presence of poor ventricular function, the more positive the effect of coronary artery bypass surgery on survival will be (e.g. in patients with left mainstem disease and triple-vessel disease).[14,15] Patients with single-vessel and two-vessel disease that does not involve the LAD obtain no survival benefit from bypass surgery compared with medical therapy, and in these patients surgery is usually reserved for intractable symptoms and failed/unsuitable angioplasty.

Reoperation

Patients who have undergone coronary artery bypass surgery may develop angina subsequently for any of the following three reasons:

1. progression of native disease;
2. graft failure;
3. a combination of (1) and (2).

Risk factor management after surgery has been shown not only to retard the progression of native coronary artery disease, but also to delay the development of graft disease, especially in vein grafts.

Newer techniques in coronary artery surgery

With the development and expansion of minimally invasive techniques in other branches of surgery, interest in this 'keyhole' approach has also evolved in the field of cardiac surgery (see Figure 11.2).

Figure 11.2
Surgery on the beating heart. An incision being made to the LAD artery with the aid of side stabilizers and an apical stabilizer, looking from the cranial position (courtesy of Miss M. Jahangiri).

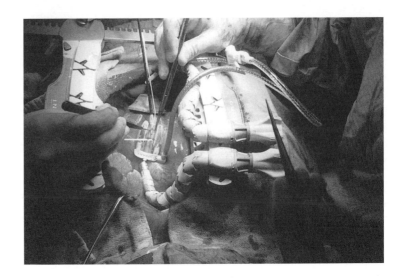

SMALLER INCISIONS

A median sternotomy incision results in a long scar, considerable post-operative pain, discomfort and slow healing. Sternal union takes approximately 3 months. It is possible to perform surgery to the front of the heart (i.e. to the LAD) using smaller incisions (e.g. a left anterior thoracotomy or a lower sternotomy).[16] The results are cosmetically superior, and because of the faster healing they result in a more rapid return to normal activities and work. They are also associated with shorter lengths of stay in hospital. The limiting factor is access to the rest of the heart (i.e. the territories of the right coronary artery and the circumflex artery).

OFF-PUMP SURGERY

Many of the complications that may follow coronary artery bypass surgery result from the use of cardiopulmonary bypass. It would be reasonable to assume, therefore, that if coronary surgery could be performed without the use of the heart–lung machine, these complications could be minimized. Off-pump surgery is usually performed using a standard median sternotomy and stabilizer devices to isolate the target coronary artery, minimize the movement of the heart, and thus facilitate accurate anastomotic technique.[17]

The limitations of off-pump surgery include the following:

- Accessing the lateral and inferior surfaces of the heart without causing haemodynamic instability, but these difficulties are being overcome.

- The problems of movement and difficult access can result in less than optimal anastomotic technique, with subsequent graft stenosis or graft failure.
- It was also thought that neurological problems would be almost eliminated by the use of off-pump surgery. However, this has not yet been shown to be the case in randomized trials. It is difficult to predict what proportion of coronary artery bypass surgery will be performed using the off-pump technique in the future. As with all of the newer techniques, the strong proponents would argue that almost every case is suitable. Conservatively, it is estimated that about 10% of all coronary cases will be performed in this way.

TRANSMYOCARDIAL REVASCULARIZATION (TMR)

This is a laser-based technique in which small channels are created in the myocardium, with potential lessening of the ischaemic burden, by either neoangiogenesis or denervation.[18] This can be performed at the time of coronary artery bypass grafting or as a stand-alone procedure in patients who are unsuitable for conventional revascularization. After initial enthusiasm, randomized trials showed a significant placebo effect, and the procedure has not been incorporated into routine clinical practice.

ANGIOGENESIS

Current research on angiogenesis is concentrating on cytokine stimulation of new vessel growth, potentially replacing fibrous tissue with revascularized myocardium.[19] These efforts have focused on patients who are unsuitable for coronary artery bypass grafting or angioplasty, and they have produced modest results in small trials. One recent study seemed to increase collateral flow in a small number of patients using granulocyte macrophage-stimulating factor to increase small-vessel proliferation.[20] Despite encouraging data from *in-vitro* work, these findings are not yet of proven clinical utility, and larger trials are awaited.

Rehabilitation

Cardiac rehabilitation has been shown to reduce mortality, increase exercise performance and improve the sense of well-being. Multidisciplinary cardiac rehabilitation programmes should be provided for all patients following coronary bypass surgery. This process can be initiated in the pre-admission clinic.

References

1. Krabatsch T, Grauham O, Hetzer R. Unilateral Vineberg arterial graft with a patency of 30 years. *Circulation* 2000; **102**: 1724–5.
2. Loop FD, Lytle BW, Cosgrove DM *et al.* Influence of internal mammary graft on 10-year survival and other cardiac events. *N Engl J Med* 1986; **314**: 1–6.
3. Treasure T. Risks and results of surgery. *Br Heart J* 1995; **74**: 1112–16.
4. Alderman EL, Bourassa M, Cohen LS *et al.* 10-year follow-up of survival and myocardial infarction in the randomized Coronary Artery Surgery Study (CASS). *Circulation* 1990; **82**: 1629–36.
5. European Coronary Surgery Study (ECSS). Randomised study of coronary artery bypass graft surgery in stable angina pectoris. *Lancet* 1980; **2**: 491–8.
6. Serruys PW, Unger F, Sousa JE *et al.* Comparison of coronary bypass surgery and stenting for the treatment of multivessel disease (ARTS). *N Engl J Med* 2001; **344**: 1117–24.
7. Pocock SJ, Henderson RA, Rickards AF *et al.* Meta-analysis of randomised trials comparing coronary angioplasty with bypass surgery. *Lancet* 1995; **346**: 1184–9.
8. Fitzgibbon GM, Kafka HB, Leach HA *et al.* Coronary bypass graft fate and patient outcome: angiographic follow-up of 5065 grafts related to survival in reoperation in 1388 patients during 25 years. *J Am Coll Cardiol* 1996; **28**: 616–26.
9. Berrekolouw E, Schonberger JP, Ercan H *et al.* Does it make sense to use two internal thoracic arteries? *Ann Thorac Surg* 1995; **59**: 1456–63.
10. Endo M, Nishada, H, Tomizov Y *et al.* Benefit of bilateral over single internal mammary artery in multiple coronary bypass grafting. *Circulation* 2001; **104**: 2164.
11. Taggart DP, D'Amicio R, Altman DG. Effect of arterial revascularisation on survival: a systematic review of studies comparing bilateral and single internal mammary arteries. *Lancet* 2001; **358**: 870–5.
12. Taggart DP, Westaby S. Neurological and cognitive disorders after coronary artery bypass grafting. *Curr Opin Cardiol* 2001; **16**: 271–6.
13. Redle JD, Khurana S, Marzan R *et al.* Prophylactic oral amiodarone compared with placebo for prevention of atrial fibrillation after coronary artery bypass surgery. *Am Heart J* 1999; **138**: 144–50.
14. Detre KM, Guo P, Holubkov R *et al.* Coronary revascularization in diabetic patients: a comparison of the randomized and observational components of the bypass angioplasty revascularization investigation (BARI). *Circulation* 1999; **99**: 633–40.
15. Espinola-Klein C, Rupprecht HJ, Erbel R *et al.* 10-year outcome after coronary angioplasty in patients with single-vessel coronary disease and

comparison with the results of the Coronary Artery Surgery Study (CASS). *Am J Cardiol* 2000; **85**: 321–6.

16. Benetti F, Mariani MA, Sani G *et al.* Video-assisted minimally invasive coronary operations without cardiopulmonary bypass: a multicentre study. *J Thorac Cardiovasc Surg* 1996; **112**: 1478–84.

17. Borst C, Jansen EW, Tulleken CA *et al.* CABG without bypass and without interruption of native coronary flow using a novel anastomosis site restraining device ('octopus'). *J Am Coll Cardiol* 1996; **27**: 1356–64.

18. Nathan M, Aranki S. Transmyocardial revascularization. *Curr Opin Cardiol* 2001; **16**: 310–14.

19. Henry TD, McKendall GR, Azrin MA *et al.* VIVA trial: one-year follow-up. *Circulation* 2000; **102** (**Supplement II**): II–1516.

20. Seiler C, Pohl T, Wustmann K *et al.* Promotion of collateral growth by GMCSF in patients with coronary artery disease. A randomized double-blind placebo-controlled trial. *Circulation* 2001; **104**: 2012.

Secondary prevention and cardiac rehabilitation

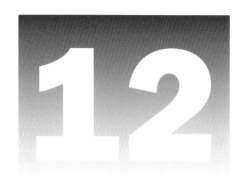

Emer Shelley

Introduction

There is strong evidence that risk of a future event can be reduced in patients with diagnosed cardiovascular disease using evidence-based treatments, including appropriate lifestyle changes.[1] When it was first started, cardiac rehabilitation focused on supervised exercise programmes to improve exercise tolerance and reduce disability after a cardiac event.[2] However, a broader approach is usually now taken, to encompass all aspects of secondary prevention, including counselling, support for behaviour change and compliance with medication.

The overall aim of secondary prevention and cardiac rehabilitation in patients with stable angina, as in patients recovering from an acute event or intervention, is to slow progression of atherosclerotic coronary disease and 'if possible induce disease regression, and reduce the risk of superimposed thrombotic complications'.[1] Patients require such preventive follow-up even if they have become asymptomatic as a result of treatment.[3] Objectives include reduction of the risk of a further non-fatal or fatal event by influencing the underlying causes of the disease. By improving patients' physical and mental health and giving attention to social conditions, they are enabled to live as full and active a life as possible. The outcome for the patient is improved quality of life as well as a longer life expectancy.

Despite widespread acceptance of the importance of secondary prevention, studies of patients in several European countries, including the UK and Ireland, have found that a substantial proportion of patients do not receive such treatments.[4] Knowledge of relevant pharmacology has not been translated into effective delivery of secondary prevention in patients with coronary heart disease (CHD). Behavioural change presents many challenges for professionals and patients. This has led to consideration of health service structures and psychological aspects of the care of patients, including those with angina.

Cardiac rehabilitation

In the UK and Ireland, the term 'cardiac rehabilitation' usually refers to a structured programme of care that commences some weeks after discharge from hospital after an acute cardiac event, an intervention or coronary artery bypass surgery. However, as emphasized in the National Service Framework (NSF) for England, cardiac rehabilitation is 'an integral component both of the acute stages of care and of secondary prevention'.[5] The need to integrate secondary prevention and cardiac rehabilitation has been recognized in the USA in the Clinical Practice Guideline entitled *Cardiac rehabilitation as secondary prevention*.[6]

Cardiac rehabilitation has been shown to improve physical function and prognosis in patients with stable angina, as well as after an acute myocardial infarction (AMI) or revascularization.[2] It has been estimated that mortality is reduced by 20–25% over 3 years when exercise training is combined with education and psychological support with a view to lifestyle modification.[7,8] However, patients with unstable angina have not been shown to benefit.

Four phases of cardiac rehabilitation have been described (see Box 12.1).[9]

Each hospital that admits patients with CHD should have systems in place to identify patients who would benefit from cardiac rehabilitation.[5] Prior to discharge from hospital, each patient should have a needs assessment for cardiac rehabilitation carried out by appropriately trained staff. The assessment should encompass medical treatment and lifestyle modification, as well as educational and psychological needs and the patient's social, vocational and family context.

There is concern in many countries about the extent to which patients are enrolled in cardiac rehabilitation programmes. This has been estimated to be only 10–20% of appropriate candidates in the USA.[2] Home-based programmes, directed by physicians and co-ordinated by nurses, have been developed to increase access to cardiac rehabilitation by patients.

The NSF acknowledges that there is under-representation in cardiac rehabilitation programmes of women, the elderly and people from ethnic minority groups. Rehabilitation programmes should consider their appropriateness for different target groups, including those on low incomes and those with physical disabilities.[5] Once trusts have an effective system for recruitment of patients after an AMI or coronary revascularization to a high-quality cardiac

Box 12.1   Four phases of cardiac rehabilitation[9]

Before discharge from hospital (phase 1)

An integral part of the acute care of someone admitted to hospital with CHD.

- Assessment of physical, psychological and social needs for cardiac rehabilitation.
- Negotiation of a written individual plan for meeting these identified needs (copies should be given to the patient and the general practitioner).
- Initial advice on lifestyle (e.g. smoking cessation, physical activity (including sexual activity), diet,[10] alcohol consumption and employment).
- Prescription of effective medication and education about its use, benefits and harmful effects.
- Involvement of relevant informal carer(s).
- Provision of information about cardiac support groups.
- Provision of locally relevant written information about cardiac rehabilitation.

Early post-discharge period (phase 2)

- Comprehensive assessment of cardiac risk, including physical, psychological and social needs for cardiac rehabilitation, and a review for the initial plan for meeting these needs.
- Provision of lifestyle advice and psychological interventions according to the agreed plan by relevant trained therapists who have access to support from a cardiologist.
- Maintain involvement of relevant informal carer(s).
- Review involvement with cardiac support groups.
- Offer resuscitation training for family members.

Four weeks after an acute cardiac event (phase 3): as phase 2 plus

- Structured exercise sessions to meet the assessed needs of individual patients.
- Maintain access to relevant advice and support from people trained to offer advice about exercise, relaxation, psychological interventions, health promotion and vocational advice.

Long-term maintenance of changed behaviour (phase 4)

- Long-term follow-up in primary care.
- Offer involvement with local cardiac support groups.
- Referral to specialist cardiac, behavioural (e.g. exercise, smoking cessation) or psychological services as clinically indicated.

rehabilitation programme, they should extend this service to patients with manifestations of CHD such as angina or heart failure.

Secondary prevention

The Second Joint Task Force of European and other Societies on Coronary Prevention summarized the factors associated with risk of a future event (see Table 12.1).[1] The Task Force recommended that in clinical practice the priority for CHD prevention should be patients with established CHD or other atherosclerotic disease. The lifestyle and therapeutic goals recommended by the Joint European Task Force have been adopted by many national planning groups.

The Clinical Standards Board for Scotland established criteria for assessing the quality of clinical services in acute hospitals for secondary prevention in patients diagnosed with AMI.[10] Many of the standards are also relevant to the care of patients with chronic stable angina. Both the Clinical Standards Board and the NSF indicate that cardiovascular status and severity of myocardial ischaemia should be assessed. With regard to risk factors, essential criteria are that the following should be assessed and documented before discharge from outpatient review to primary care:

- smoking history;
- cholesterol measurement;
- blood pressure measurement;

Table 12.1
Lifestyles and characteristics associated with increased risk of future CHD[1]

Lifestyle	Biochemical or physiological characteristics modifiable	Personal characteristics (non-modifiable)
Diet high in saturated fat, cholesterol and calories Tobacco smoking Excess alcohol consumption Physical inactivity	Elevated blood pressure Elevated plasma total cholesterol (LDL-cholesterol) levels Low plasma HDL-cholesterol levels Elevated plasma triglyceride levels Hyperglycaemia/diabetes Obesity Thrombogenic factors	Age Sex Family history of CHD or other atherosclerotic disease at early age (in men < 55 years, in women < 65 years) Personal history of CHD or other atherosclerotic vascular disease

- history of alcohol consumption;
- body mass index;
- blood glucose measurement;
- history of physical activity.

The recommendations of the NSF with regard to the management of patients with stable angina are very similar to those of the European Task Force.[11] After investigations into aetiology and assessment of risk, the NSF divided the treatment of patients with angina into medications for the relief of symptoms and treatment (including lifestyle advice) to improve prognosis (see Box 12.2). The NSF patient target for diastolic blood pressure is lower (at 85 mmHg) than that set by the European Task Force (95 mmHg). The NSF recognizes the target as challenging but appropriate. It is acknowledged that in practice it will not be possible to achieve this for every patient, but that practitioners should not be satisfied with pressures of greater than 150 mmHg systolic or 90 mmHg diastolic in these high-risk patients.

The targets for blood cholesterol levels are also qualified in the NSF. As in the European recommendations, the targets are set at 5 mmol/L (total

---

Box 12.2   Medical therapies for patients with chronic stable angina, as summarized in the National Service Framework for England (2000)[11]

Treatment to relieve symptoms

- Sublingual nitrates for immediate symptom control.
- Beta-blockers and/or nitrates and/or calcium antagonists.

Treatment to reduce cardiovascular risk

- Advice about how to stop smoking (including advice about the use of nicotine replacement therapy).
- Information about other modifiable risk factors, and personalized advice about how they can be reduced (this includes advice about physical activity, diet, weight, alcohol consumption and diabetes).
- Advice and treatment for maintaining blood pressure below 140/85 mmHg.
- Low-dose aspirin (75 mg daily).
- Statins and dietary advice to lower serum cholesterol concentrations *either* to less than 5 mmol/L (LDL-cholesterol to below 3 mmol/L or by 30%, whichever is greater).
- Education about symptoms of heart attack and, should they develop, instruction to seek help rapidly.

cholesterol) and 3 mmol/L (LDL-cholesterol), but the NSF adds an alternative goal, namely to lower cholesterol measurements by 30% if that represents greater reductions. The mechanism of action of medications that have been shown to be effective in the long-term care of patients with coronary artery disease, their contraindications and side-effects are described in Chapter 9.

Risk reduction in patients with diabetes

It is accepted that the management of cardiovascular risk factors is essential in patients with diabetes even before the onset of symptoms.[12] The UK Prospective Diabetes Study (UKPDS) found that in patients with type 2 diabetes the risk of diabetic complications was strongly associated with previous hyperglycaemia, including risk of AMI and of microvascular complications.[13] The risk was lowest in those with HbA_{1c} in the normal range (<6.0%). Risk of diabetic complications was also strongly associated with raised blood pressure.[14] The lowest risk was found in those with systolic blood pressure below 120 mmHg. Diabetics with diagnosed vascular disease are at particularly high risk of recurrence. A study in Finland found that 45.0% of patients with diabetes and a history of myocardial infarction at baseline had a recurrence of myocardial infarction during 7 years of follow-up, compared with 20.2% of diabetics without such a history.[15] For patients who were not diabetic, the corresponding incidence figures were 18.8% and 3.5%, respectively.

Patients with diabetes and cardiovascular disease have been shown to benefit from interventions to reduce risk. The Scandinavian Simvastatin Survival Study (4S) showed that the reduction in coronary events was even greater in patients with diabetes than in those without the condition (55% and 32%, respectively).[16] The International Diabetes Federation summarized the findings as follows: 'in the diabetes group there was a saving of one life for every four patients treated, as opposed to one in 13 in the group of people without the disease.'[12] Evidence from other studies, such as the Cholesterol and Recurrent Events (CARE) trial, supports lipid-lowering in patients with type 2 diabetes, particularly if they already have CHD.[17]

Thus risk reduction should be pursued aggressively in asymptomatic diabetic patients, but particularly in diabetics with diagnosed vascular disease, including angina. There is evidence from randomized controlled trials as well as from observational studies that in both types of diabetes the aim should be for the best glucose control which can be achieved in order to reduce the risk of CHD and other atherosclerotic disease. Advice with regard to diet, physical activity, smoking cessation and reduction of overweight is similar to that for reduction of risk of cardiovascular disease in general.[1] In addition, the Joint

European Task Force recommends that risk-factor goals should be more ambitious in patients with diabetes than in non-diabetics.

- For blood pressure lowering, <130/85 mmHg is the primary goal and a lower level is desirable in patients with diabetic nephropathy.
- In isolated systolic hypertension, usually elderly patients with type 2 diabetes, the goal for patients with a systolic blood pressure of >180 mmHg is <160 mmHg, and for patients with a systolic blood pressure of 160–179 mmHg, the primary goal is a reduction of 20 mmHg. If these goals are achieved and well tolerated, then further lowering to 140 mmHg may be appropriate.
- Elevated triglycerides and low HDL-cholesterol levels are markers of excess risk in patients with type 2 diabetes. The International Federation of Diabetes (Europe) recommends that in patients with diabetes, the target HDL-cholesterol level is >1.2 mmol/L, and the target for triglycerides is <1.7 mmol/L.[12]
- The minimum goal for LDL-cholesterol levels in diabetic patients with CHD is <3.0 mmol/L, although the American Diabetes Association has recommended that the goal should be <2.6 mmol/L in patients with any atherosclerotic vascular disease. In those without CHD, the goal is <3.0 mmol/L.

Smoking cessation

It is cause for concern that many studies of patients with diagnosed CHD confirm a continuing smoking prevalence of 20% or higher.[18] There is substantial evidence that stopping smoking reduces the risk of cardiovascular disease.[19] Following myocardial infarction, one study showed that the risk of a non-fatal recurrence and of cardiovascular death was halved in those who quit smoking. A UK trial in smokers with evidence of CHD found a 13% difference (statistically non-significant) in CHD deaths over 20 years in those who were given cessation advice compared to those who were not given such advice.

Smoking interventions in clinical practice have been summarized as follows:[19,20]

- *Assess* the smoking status of the patient – non-smoker, ex-smoker or smoker.
- *Advise* all smokers of the importance of stopping from a health perspective, especially in the case of those who already have a smoking-related disease.
- *Assist* smokers in stopping, especially those with smoking-related disease and those who express an interest in stopping.
- *Arrange* follow-up.

It is accepted that very brief advice by a clinician to stop smoking is effective in increasing the percentage of smokers who stop and remain abstinent at 6 months.[20] One of the main effects of brief advice is to motivate patients to attempt to quit, but many need more specialist advice and support to stop smoking and to maintain the new behaviour. This applies especially to heavier smokers, who are more at risk of smoking-related disease.

Physician advice during hospital admission with AMI, together with nurse-managed intervention during hospitalization, have shown improved smoking cessation outcomes.[2] To prevent relapse after discharge, the patient can be provided with behavioural skills for coping in high-risk situations, relaxation training, and maintenance of telephone contact after discharge, as well as bupropion or nicotine replacement therapy (NRT) as appropriate. The former drug has been associated with arrhythmias, especially in overdose, and must be used with caution.

Patients in the community can be referred to a smoking cessation specialist.[20] Whenever possible, support should be provided in a group setting. Social support and training in coping skills are provided in five 1-hour sessions over a period of 4 weeks, with longer-term follow-up being offered. Patients should be offered NRT with clear instructions on how to use it.

NRT (in the form of gum, patches, nasal spray or inhaler) was developed to provide a temporary alternative source of nicotine to allay withdrawal symptoms.[19] Placebo-controlled trials have shown that, when used in conjunction with advice from a health professional, NRT can double quit rates compared with placebo. The evidence is particularly strong for nicotine gum and nicotine patches. Cessation rates of 20% in the NRT groups compare with rates of approximately 10% in the control group.

Nicotine patches have been tested in patients with CHD without adverse effects.[1] However, the Joint European Task Force advises caution in the use of NRT in these patients. In particular, patients should be warned not to smoke while using NRT.

Diet and dyslipidaemia

Nutrition education is an essential component of secondary prevention in all patients with diagnosed atherosclerotic vascular disease.[1] The dietetic goals are similar to those for the general population, with modification of fat intake and increased consumption of fresh fruits, vegetables and cereals. The goal for fat intake in patients with a vascular disease is lower than that for the general population, at 30% or less of total energy intake.[1] The goal for total cholesterol intake is 300 mg/day, although this is mainly achieved through attention to total fat intake and to the type and ratio of fats consumed. Saturated fats should represent one-third of total fat intake, and must be replaced in part with monounsaturated and polyunsaturated fats from both vegetable and marine sources.

It is estimated that a reduction in dietary saturated fat equivalent to 10% of calories will lower serum total cholesterol levels by about 1 mmol/L, with projected long-term reductions in CHD mortality of 40%.[21] *Trans*-unsaturated fatty acids have also been shown to increase serum total and LDL-cholesterol levels by about as much as long-chain saturated fatty acids. *Trans*-fats are generated during the process of hydrogenating oils to produce hard margarines. Naturally occurring *cis*-unsaturated fatty acids reduce serum cholesterol levels by about half as much as longer-chain saturated fatty acids increase it.

In reviewing evidence about dietary management, the North of England Evidence-Based Guideline Development Project on the management of patients with stable angina stated that 'patients who have survived a myocardial infarction and take a "Mediterranean diet" or increase their intake of fatty fish have a lower rate of subsequent cardiovascular events'.[22] The subjects in the trials had survived an AMI, but such trials have not been conducted in patients with stable angina who have not had an AMI. The accompanying recommendation of a Mediterranean diet and twice-weekly oily fish relates to patients with stable angina who have survived a myocardial infarction. Even in the absence of clinical trials, it seems nonsensical to confine advice about eating vegetables and oily fish to symptomatic patients who have survived an AMI. The NSF supports a more proactive approach, referring to the trial of Mediterranean diet after AMI in support of its recommendation that those at high risk of a future cardiovascular event should receive dietary advice.[23]

The Clinical Standards Board for Scotland recommends that after an AMI, patients whose total cholesterol level is above 6 mmol/L should be treated with a statin, in accordance with Scottish guidelines.[10] However, patients whose cholesterol level is between 5 and 6 mmol/L should be managed with dietary advice for 3 months before the introduction of a statin. The pharmacological management of raised lipids is described in Chapter 9 (p. 123).

Weight loss

There is widespread agreement that patients who are at high risk of a future cardiovascular disease event, including those with diagnosed disease, should be advised to lose weight. The North of England Evidence-Based Guideline Development Project report on the management of stable angina concluded that there is strong evidence that 'hypertensive patients with a body mass index (BMI) above the normal range should be encouraged to reduce their body weight until their body mass index (BMI) is as close to normal as is achievable.'[22] The project also recommends, although on a weaker evidence base, that normotensive patients with stable angina should be similarly encouraged to aim for normal BMI.

The NSF and the Joint European Task Force recommend appropriate weight reduction in those identified as being at high risk of a cardiovascular disease event.[1,23] The Task Force acknowledges that 'reduction of overweight is not easy'. In addition to motivation of the individual, encouragement and long-term support by the physician are required. Realistic goals should be agreed between the patients and their physicians (e.g. 0.5 to 1.0 kg per week). Patients require counselling in the practical aspects of weight reduction using an energy-restricted, lipid-lowering diet. Regular physical activity aids both weight reduction and weight maintenance.

Physical activity

For most patients with angina, resumption of normal activities is an important goal of treatment.[3] In addition to medication aimed at symptom relief, 'education and exercise' are an integral component of treatment strategies. It has been concluded that exercise rehabilitation contributes to symptom relief in angina.[6] The evidence in support of exercise training programmes has been classified as intermediate, on a par with the evidence for the effectiveness of smoking cessation or lipid lowering.[3] However, it is difficult to separate out the benefits of exercise training *per se* from the beneficial effects of activity on other risk variables (e.g. weight reduction, improved lipid profiles and lower blood pressure).

Early cardiac rehabilitation programmes provided standard exercise regimes for all.[2] Nowadays, exercise is prescribed as appropriate to the person's clinical profile, including their age, functional status and other risk factors. For most patients, some form of aerobic exercise is recommended, such as walking or cycling. Those under 65 years of age should aim for an intensity of 75–85% of maximal heart rate, in sessions of 30–45 min, three to four times a week. For those over 65 years, the recommendation is for a maximal heart rate of 65–75% for 30 min per session, together with resistance training.

Patients who are overweight should aim for high caloric expenditure, walking at 65–80% of maximal heart rate for longer periods and more frequently (e.g. five or six times weekly for 45 to 60 min).[2] Resistance training should be prescribed for those over 65 years of age and those who are disabled or overweight. Using weight machines and dumb-bells, with the focus on the upper legs, shoulders and arms, sessions should be at an intensity of 50–70% at a single repetition of what can be achieved at maximal lift, for 10–20 min in total across a range of exercises, two or three times a week.

Blood pressure

The association between blood pressure and risk of a cerebrovascular or CHD event has been shown to be positive and continuous.[24] No lower level has been identified below which the risks do not continue to decline. The risk of heart failure and renal disease is also related to blood pressure. It has been estimated that a sustained lowering of blood pressure by 5 mmHg lowers the risk of these adverse outcomes by between one-third and one-quarter. The increased risk of a future major cardiovascular event in patients with diagnosed vascular disease strengthens the case for attention to blood pressure in patients with stable or unstable angina.

Some factors that affect the risk of cardiovascular disease do so through their effects on blood pressure.[24] The increased risk of CHD associated with being overweight or obese is likely to be due in part to raised blood pressure, although lower HDL-cholesterol and increased insulin and glucose levels are also relevant. Some of the benefits of being physically active on a regular basis are mediated through lower blood pressure levels.

The association between alcohol intake and risk of CHD is complex, with regular moderate consumption (1–3 drinks a day) being associated with a 30–40% lower risk of CHD death compared with non-drinkers. However, high alcohol consumption raises blood pressure levels and increases the risk of stroke (particularly after binge drinking), in addition to being associated with cardio-myopathy and other non-vascular conditions, including injury. As well as lowering blood pressure, alcohol intake and physical activity are associated with increased HDL-cholesterol levels, contributing to their risk-lowering potential.

Although the lifestyle and behavioural factors associated with raised blood pressure present many challenges, the benefits of complementary pharmaco-logical therapy are accepted, to achieve the targets as set out above. The pharmacology of antihypertensive agents is described in Chapter 9 (p. 117). Despite the many agents now on the market, with much fewer side-effects than in the early days of such treatment, it is apparent that many patients with diagnosed cardiovascular disease have raised blood pressure which is either being inadequately treated or not being treated at all.[4] Effective risk reduction for all patients requires comprehensive patient education and coun-selling. In addition, health service structures need to be put in place to ensure consistency and continuity of care, particularly at the interface between acute hospitals and primary care, including general practice.

Supporting behaviour change

When the link was first made between particular behaviours and illness, it was naively believed that, once they had been made aware of the association, individuals would abandon the habit in favour of the healthier alternative. However, it became apparent that it is very challenging to change the behaviour of a lifetime. When a diagnosis of CHD is made, the patient may then be more motivated to change, but many struggle to make changes and require the support of trained professionals.

A number of theories of behaviour change have been used to try to understand why people maintain particular health behaviours. Health professionals can apply these theories when supporting individuals to develop new behaviour patterns.

The *health belief model* attempts to explain and predict health behaviours by focusing on the attitudes and beliefs of individuals.[25] Key variables of the model include the following:

- perceived threat, including perceived susceptibility and beliefs about the severity of the condition;
- perceived benefits – beliefs about the effectiveness of strategies to reduce the risk;
- perceived barriers – beliefs about the potential negative effects of a health action, including the physical, psychological and financial prerequisites;
- cues to action (this may include the onset of symptoms);
- self-efficacy – the belief in one's capacity to sustain the required action and to achieve the desired outcome.

The *theory of reasoned action* is based on the premise that human beings are rational and that the behaviour of interest can be determined by the individual. The theoretical framework links the individual's beliefs, attitudes, intentions and behaviour. The behaviour is described on the basis of the required action, the target to be attained, the context in which the behaviour is to be applied and the planned frequency of the action. The basic premise is that the individual's beliefs about the behaviour, including their perceptions about society's beliefs, influence their attitudes and intentions, which in turn influence behaviour and outcomes.[26]

The *stages of change* model is widely used as a basis for brief intervention for behaviour change (see Box 12.3). The stages are components of a cyclical process of behaviour change.[27] Processes at each stage help to predict and motivate the person's movement across the stages, although change does not necessarily occur in a linear fashion from one stage to the next. Identification of the stage of the individual in the cycle enables the health professional to provide appropriate advice and support. Programme evaluation can measure the extent to which individuals move through the change process.

The stages of change model has been criticized because it focuses on the individual, with limited attention being paid to the broader environmental issues that impact on the person's ability to change. However, it can be difficult

> **Box 12.3 Stages of change model: the stages of behaviour and processes of change**[27]
>
> **Precontemplation**
>
> Individual practises the 'problem' behaviour and has no intention of changing.
>
> *Processes:* Consciousness raising (information and knowledge).
> Dramatic exploration and role play.
> Environmental evaluation (how problem affects physical environment).
>
> **Contemplation**
>
> Individual recognizes the problem and is seriously thinking about changing.
>
> *Process:* Self-evaluation (assessing one's feelings with regard to the behaviour).
>
> **Preparation for action**
>
> Individual recognizes the problem and intends to change within the next month. May report some inconsistent behaviour change efforts.
>
> *Process:* Self-liberation (commitment or belief in ability to change).
>
> **Action**
>
> Individual has been carrying out new behaviour for less than 6 months.
>
> *Processes:* Reinforcement and rewards.
> Social support and self-help groups.
> Counter-conditioning and alternatives for behaviour.
> Stimulus control, avoiding high-risk cues.
>
> **Maintenance**
>
> Individual maintains the new behaviour for 6 months or more.

and time-consuming to change public policy or to bring about organizational change, so the focus on empowering the individual to adopt new health behaviours can also be viewed as one of the strengths of the stages of change theory for use by health professionals.

It is recognized that behaviour within society at large influences the behaviour of individuals.[28] Bandura's social cognitive theory places an emphasis on self-efficacy, set in the context of societal incentives and disincentives to health behaviours. From a public health perspective, most lives are saved by a modest reduction in risk in the majority of the population in the middle and even the lower end of the risk distribution – 'the population approach'. From a clinical perspective, those individuals who are at high absolute risk of a future event, including those who are symptomatic, have the most to gain from action to reduce their level of risk.

Farquhar called for a broadened set of actions by health-care professionals, including advocacy for political action and public education, with an emphasis on precursors to risk factors.[28] Regulatory and environmental barriers to change include access to healthy food choices (e.g. in schools and colleges), and the availability of safe and convenient facilities for walking or other forms of physical activity. Most professionals are likely to contribute in only a minor way to bringing about environmental and societal change. However, all of them should be aware of the challenges that their patients face in adopting healthy lifestyles in societies where smoking is commonplace and obesity and physical inactivity are on the increase.

Compliance

The term compliance refers to the extent to which recommendations are followed as defined.[29] The American Heart Association's Expert Panel refers to the 'multilevel compliance challenge'. This encompasses not just the patient's behavioural response to advice, but also the actions of health professionals and strategies utilized by health-care organizations that contribute to improving the effective application of clinical guidelines. It is recognized that the evidence base for specific strategies to improve compliance is not strong. However, there is evidence that strategies such as self-monitoring and telephone follow-up may improve compliance, and multicomponent strategies have been shown to be effective.

Health professionals can support compliance through effective communications, using clear messages and negotiating treatment plans and goals with patients.[29] Barriers to compliance can be anticipated and potential solutions discussed. Progress in achieving goals should be assessed at each visit.

Health-care organizations can support the translation of scientific knowledge into effective clinical practice through education and training for professionals and through supportive health-care structures (e.g. systems for telephone follow-up, and computerized patient-tracking systems to arrange follow-up and record progress). Management should support co-ordinated input from all team members, including nurse specialists and pharmacists. The American Heart Association Panel concluded that the incorporation of current knowledge into a multilevel approach offers enormous potential for decreasing risk and improving patient outcomes.

In conclusion, cardiac rehabilitation is a multifaceted approach to the patient recovering from a cardiac event, incorporating exercise, diet, lipid and psychosocial programmes, and it involves secondary prevention as a key component of any doctor–patient interface.

References

1. Wood D, De Backer G, Faergeman O *et al.* Prevention of coronary heart disease in clinical practice. Recommendations of the Second Joint Task Force of European and other Societies on Coronary Prevention. *Eur Heart J* 1998; **19**: 1434–503.

2. Ades PA. Cardiac rehabilitation and secondary prevention of coronary heart disease. *N Engl J Med* 2001; **345**: 892–902.

3. Gibbons RJU, Chatterjee K, Daley J *et al.* American College of Cardiology/American Heart Association Task Force on Practice Guidelines (Committee on Management of Patients with Chronic Stable Angina). ACC/AHA/ACP-ASIM guidelines for the management of patients with chronic stable angina: executive summary and recommendations. *Circulation* 1999; **99**: 2829–48.

4. EUROASPIRE II Study Group. Lifestyle and risk factor management and use of drug therapies in coronary patients from 15 countries: principal results from EUROASPIRE II Euro Heart Survey Programme. *Eur Heart J* 2001; **22**: 554–72.

5. Department of Health. Cardiac rehabilitation. *NHS. Our Healthier Nation.* In: *National Service Frameworks. Coronary heart disease.* London: Department of Health, 2000: 1–29, Chapter 7.

6. Wenger NK, Froelicher ES, Smith LK *et al. Cardiac rehabilitation as secondary prevention.* Clinical Practice Guideline. Quick Reference Guide for Clinicians No. 17. Rockville, MD: US Department of Health and Human Services, Public Health Service, Agency for Health Care Policy and Research and National Heart, Lung, and Blood Institute, 1995.

7. Oldridge NB, Guyatt GH, Fisher ME, Rimm AA. Cardiac rehabilitation after myocardial infarction: combined experience of randomized clinical trials. *J Am Med Assoc* 1988; **260**: 945–50.

8. O'Connor GT, Buring GE, Yusuf S *et al.* An overview of randomized trials of rehabilitation with exercise after myocardial infarction. *Circulation* 1989; **80**: 234–44.

9. Horgan JH, Bethell H, Carson P *et al.* British Cardiac Society Working Group on Cardiac Rehabilitation. *Br Heart J* 1992; **67**: 412–18.

10. Clinical Standards Board for Scotland. *Clinical standards. Secondary prevention following acute myocardial infarction.* Edinburgh: Clinical Standards Board for Scotland, 2000.

11. Department of Health. Stable angina. In: *NHS. Our Healthier Nation. National Service Framework. Coronary heart disease.* London: Department of Health, 2000: 1–24, Chapter 4.

12. International Diabetes Federation and Cardiovascular Disease Editorial Committee. *Diabetes and cardiovascular disease. Time to act.* Brussels: International Diabetes Federation, 2001.

13. Stratton IM, Adler AI, Neil AW *et al.* Association of glycaemia with macrovascular and microvascular complications of type 2 diabetes (UKPDS 35): prospective observational study. *Br Med J* 2000; **321**: 405–12.

14. Adler AI, Stratton IM, Neil AW *et al.* Association of systolic blood pressure with macrovascular and microvascular complications of type 2 diabetes (UKPDS 36): prospective observational study. *Br Med J* 2000; **321**: 412–19.

15. Haffner SM, Lehto S, Ronnemaa T, Pyorala K, Laakso M. Mortality from coronary heart disease in subjects with type 2 diabetes and in non-diabetic subjects with and without prior myocardial infarction. *N Engl J Med* 1998; **339**: 229–34.

16. Scandinavian Simvastatin Survival Study Group. Randomised trial of cholesterol lowering in 4444 patients with coronary heart disease: the Scandinavian Simvastatin Survival Study (4S). *Lancet* 1994; **344**: 1383–9.

17. Goldberg RB, Mellies MJ, Sacks FM *et al.* Cardiovascular events and their reduction with pravastatin in diabetic and glucose-intolerant myocardial infarction survivors with average cholesterol levels: sub-group analyses in the Cholesterol and Recurrent Events (CARE) trial. *Circulation* 1998; **98**: 2513–19.

18. EUROASPIRE I and II Group. Clinical reality of coronary prevention guidelines: a comparison of EUROASPIRE I and II in nine countries. *Lancet* 2001; **357**: 995–1001.

19. Fowler G. Tobacco and cardiovascular disease: achieving smoking cessation. In: Yusuf S, Cairns JA, Camm AJ, Fallen EL, Gersh BJ (eds) *Evidence-based cardiology*. London: BMJ Books, 1998: 179–90.

20. Raw M, McNeill A, West R. Smoking cessation: evidence-based recommendations for the healthcare system. *Br Med J* 1999; **318**: 182–5.

21. Law M. Lipids and cardiovascular disease. In: Yusuf S, Cairns JA, Camm AJ, Fallen EL, Gersh BJ (eds) *Evidence-based cardiology*. London: BMJ Books, 1998: 191–205.

22. Eccles M, Rousseau N, Adam P *et al.* North of England Stable Angina Development Group. *Fam Pract* 2001; **18**: 217–22.

23. Department of Health. Preventing coronary heart disease in high-risk patients. *NHS. Our Healthier Nation.* In: *National Service Frameworks. Coronary heart disease.* London: Department of Health, 2000: 1–45, Chapter 2.

24. Guidelines Subcommittee. World Health Organisation – International Society of Hypertension Guidelines for the Management of Hypertension. *J Hypertens* 1999; **17**: 151–83.

25. Rosenstock L, Strecher V, Becker M. The health belief model and HIV risk behavior change. In: DiClemente RJ, Peterson JL (eds) *Preventing*

AIDS: theories and methods of behavioral interventions. New York: Plenum Press, 1994: 5–24.

26. Fishbein M, Middlestadt SE, Hitchcock PJ. Using information to change sexually transmitted disease-related behaviours. In: DiClemente RJ, Peterson JL (eds) *Preventing AIDS: theories and methods of behavioral interventions.* New York: Plenum Press, 1994: 61–78.

27. Prochaska JO, DiClemente CC, Norcross JC. In search of how people change – applications to addictive behaviors. *Am Psychol* 1992; **47**: 1102–14.

28. Farquhar JW. Keynote address: how health behavior relates to risk factors. American Heart Association Prevention Conference III on behaviour change and compliance: keys to improving cardiovascular health, 15–17 January 1993, Monterey, California. *Circulation* 1993; **88**: 1376–80.

29. Houston Miller N, Hill M, Kottke T, Ockene IS for the Expert Panel on Compliance. The multilevel compliance challenge: recommendations for a call to action. A statement for healthcare professionals. *Circulation* 1997; **95**: 1085–90.

Health economic aspects of angina

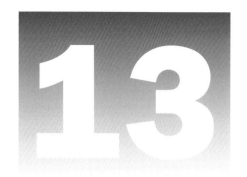

Michael Barry and John Feely

Introduction

Cardiovascular disease is the leading source of health-care expenditure in the USA and most other industrialized countries. It accounted for $274 billion in US medical spending and lost output in 1998. The 5-year cost of coronary artery disease has been estimated to be $50 000 per case.[1] With regard to angina pectoris, it has been estimated that the prevalence ranges from 30 000 to 40 000 per million members of the population in countries with high coronary heart disease rates, such as Ireland. This prevalence increases with age to approximately 15% of men and 12% of women in the 65–74-years age group. A Swedish study has calculated that the annual direct medical costs (i.e. all costs occurring within the health sector, including hospitalization, health-care professional costs, medications, laboratory tests and procedures) for angina pectoris consumed approximately 3% of the health-care budget.[2] In a recent study in the USA, direct medical costs for stable and unstable angina pectoris were estimated to be $2569 and $12 058 per patient per annum, respectively.[3]

Factors that contribute to the cost of angina pectoris

In 1995, Andersson et al.[2] identified the variables with the greatest impact on direct medical costs of angina pectoris in Sweden. The study included information obtained from 402 general practitioners. The direct medical cost of angina per patient was estimated to be $3756. The greatest contribution to this cost was hospitalization (45%), with drug therapy accounting for 6% of the total cost. Laboratory investigations and the procedures of coronary artery bypass grafting (CABG) and percutaneous transluminal coronary angioplasty (PTCA) accounted for 12.4% and 12.5% of costs, respectively.

Direct medical costs peaked in patients aged 51–60 years, and were reduced in older age groups. This may be related to increased mortality among patients with severe angina pectoris over time. The number of investigations, procedures and hospitalizations was greater in male patients, resulting in higher costs. Men with angina were on average 6 years younger, and were more likely to have had cardiovascular surgery. The severity of angina was related to the associated costs, as annual expenditure on patients with four or more angina episodes per week was approximately 20% higher than that on patients with fewer than four episodes per week. Expenditure relating to patients with unstable angina pectoris was over twofold higher than that for patients who had stable angina. The increased expenditure for severe angina was primarily related to hospitalization rates. The study showed that the longer the time period since the first diagnosis of angina, the lower the direct medical costs. Not surprisingly, those patients who underwent PTCA and CABG had increased costs ($6434 and $2922, respectively). Annual non-medical costs, including travel, means of assistance, extra home care, employment issues or early retirement pension, amounted to $3585 (i.e. similar to direct medical expenditure). As expected, non-medical costs were higher for patients under 65 years of age than for patients over 65 years. The annual direct medical cost per patient for angina pectoris was similar to that for myocardial infarction.

Therefore the significant variables contributing to the direct costs of angina pectoris included the following:

1. cardiovascular surgery;
2. treatment in the general practice or hospital setting;
3. the number of years since the first diagnosis of angina;
4. whether the patient's angina was characterized as stable or unstable.

Diagnosis of angina pectoris

The cost-effectiveness of different diagnostic strategies for patients with chest pain has been analysed by Kuntz et al.[4] on the assumption that patients can perform an exercise stress test. The choices were as follows:

1. no testing and medical treatment as appropriate;
2. exercise electrocardiogram (ECG) (US$110) with coronary angiography ($4741) if test is positive;

3. exercise echocardiography ($262) with coronary angiography if tests are positive;
4. exercise single photon emission computed tomography (SPECT) ($574) with coronary angiography if tests are positive;
5. routine coronary angiography without previous non-invasive testing.

For patients with a very low probability of coronary heart disease, the cost-effectiveness ratio of all testing strategies was higher than that of other well-accepted medical interventions. The use of non-invasive testing is associated with reasonable cost-effectiveness ratios for patients at moderate risk for coronary disease. The choice of non-invasive tests, exercise ECG, ECHO or SPECT depends on institution-specific estimates of sensitivity and specificity. The incremental cost-effectiveness ratio (i.e. the amount of additional benefit for the additional cost) of routine coronary angiography compared with exercise echocardiography was $36 400 per quality-adjusted life year (QALY) gained for a 55-year-old man with typical angina. For a 55-year-old man with non-specific chest pain, the incremental cost-effectiveness ratio of exercise electrocardiography compared with no testing was $57 700 per QALY gained. It was concluded that coronary angiography without previous non-invasive testing should be reserved for patients who have a very high probability of disease and who present with severe symptoms of typical angina.

For women who are referred for diagnostic evaluation of stable chest pain, stress myocardial perfusion imaging followed by selective angiography in those patients with at least one perfusion abnormally minimizes the near-term composite costs per patient compared with a direct referral for angiography, regardless of the pre-test likelihood of coronary heart disease.[5]

In another study, patients with chest pain who were referred to a cardiologist from a gatekeeper-managed care organization were compared with those who were referred from an open-access managed care organization.[6] Although the type of cardiology services provided did not differ, in the latter system many more patients saw a cardiologist. Furthermore, they were likely to continue to be seen by a cardiologist. The rates of cardiac catheterization procedures and hospitalization were similar. The lower volume of referrals and co-ordination of care suggest potential cost advantages for the gatekeeper model.

Drug treatment of angina pectoris

Aspirin significantly reduces the risk of myocardial infarction in patients with a history of stable or unstable angina pectoris, and reduces the risk of death in patients with a history of stable angina pectoris.[7,8] Regardless of the perspective considered (direct medical costs, social security or societal perspectives), the use of the cost-effectiveness ratio at 1 year for the prevention of myocardial infarction and death in patients with a history of unstable angina has been demonstrated to be a cost-saving strategy, as the benefits of prophylaxis exceeded the costs. For example, the savings that result from the reduction of myocardial infarction following treatment of patients with unstable angina pectoris with aspirin, 75 mg per day, have been estimated to be $4633 in relation to direct medical costs, and $8576 from the societal perspective.[9] In patients with stable angina pectoris, a 4-year follow-up has shown that aspirin, 75 mg per day, as prophylaxis was associated with additional direct medical costs of $4752 and $4273 per event avoided (i.e. myocardial infarction and death, respectively). If the societal perspective was adopted, the additional costs would be estimated to be $720 and $646, respectively.[9]

Platelet glycoprotein IIb–IIIa receptor antagonists

Unlike antiplatelet agents that target only one of many individual pathways involved in platelet aggregation, antagonists of glycoprotein IIb–IIIa maximally inhibit the final common pathway involved in platelet adhesion, activation and aggregation. There are three classes of glycoprotein IIb–IIIa inhibitors, which include murine–human chimeric antibodies (abciximab), synthetic peptide forms (eptifibatide) and synthetic non-peptide forms (tirofiban).[10] For the 3230 patients with unstable angina pectoris who were enrolled with the PRISM trial, the platelet glycoprotein IIb–IIIa receptor antagonist tirofiban demonstrated a reduction in clinical end-points. Heeschen et al.[11] investigated the cost-effectiveness of tirofiban according to a reduction in cardiac events (death, acute myocardial infarction), necessity for coronary intervention and duration of hospitalization. For acute myocardial infarction, an absolute difference of 1.3% at 30 days (94.2% vs. 92.9%, tirofiban vs. heparin) was noted. The incremental cost-effectiveness was estimated to be $68 062.[11] In general, a therapeutic intervention that has a cost-effectiveness ratio of $50 000 or less per year of life saved is considered to be cost-effective. More favourable results were obtained from the limited use of tirofiban in high-risk patients with elevated troponin levels. For troponin-I-positive patients, the absolute difference in acute myocardial infarction at 30 days was 8.7%. The associated costs for troponin-I-positive patients were lower for those treated with tirofiban than for those treated with heparin ($8613 vs. $9197), with an incremental cost-effectiveness of $8941.[11] Similar results were obtained from troponin-T analysis. The authors concluded that treatment with platelet glycoprotein IIb–IIIa receptor antagonists in patients with acute coronary syndromes was only cost-effective in troponin-positive patients. Houghton et al.[12] investigated the cost implications of introducing tirofiban for the treatment of acute coronary syndromes in the coronary care unit. Treating patients who satisfied the entry criteria for the PRISM-Plus study resulted in additional drug costs of £85 for every admission with unstable angina or non-Q-wave myocardial infarction. A non-evidence-based approach that involved treating all such patients resulted in additional drug costs estimated at £342 for every admission.[12] The authors highlighted the importance of an evidence-based protocol to ensure the cost-effectiveness of the drug. Cost–benefit analyses of recent studies are awaited.

Anti-thrombotic therapy

Unlike unfractionated heparin, preparations of low-molecular-weight heparin have in common a predictable pharmacokinetic profile, high bioavailability, a long plasma half-life and an easy means of administration (subcutaneous injection) without the need to monitor activated partial thromboplastin time. However, low-molecular-weight heparins are considerably more expensive than unfractionated heparin, and therefore the question of cost-effectiveness arises. Detournay *et al.* conducted an economic evaluation of enoxaparin sodium vs. heparin in patients with unstable angina pectoris and non-Q-wave myocardial infarction.[13] This study was conducted from the societal perspective. The primary efficacy parameter in the ESSENCE trial was a composite end-point of the incidence of death, non-fatal myocardial infarction and recurrent angina measured 14 days after randomization. Enoxaparin therapy reduced the incidence of the primary end-point by 16.2%. Among patients treated with enoxaparin, there was a significant reduction in the use of angiography and PTCA, which produced cost savings estimated to be $143 per treated patient. Analysis based on the duration of hospital stay resulted in estimated savings of $113 per treated patient. A one-way sensitivity analysis indicated that the difference in procedure rates was mainly sensitive to the lower PTCA rate. With regard to the length of stay, intensive-care unit daily costs were of particular importance. Economic studies based on US and UK patient subgroups also demonstrated cost savings of $1165 and £23.00, respectively, per patient.[14,15] Variations in procedure costs account for much of the difference in estimated cost savings in the different countries. The US economic analysis of the ESSENCE trial identified five main cost drivers, namely coronary angiography, PTCA, CABG, length of stay in an intensive-care unit, and the length of non-intensive-care unit hospitalization.

Lipid-lowering therapy

Cholesterol lowering by pharmacological intervention prevents the progression of atherosclerosis and reduces both fatal and non-fatal coronary events in patients with or without coronary artery disease. Initial cost-effectiveness studies of non-statin interventions (e.g. bile acid resins, niacin, diet and fibric acid derivatives) indicated that such strategies would only be cost-effective in high-risk patients.[16] For the bile acid resin cholestyramine, studies indicated that it is not cost-effective except in patients aged 35–45 years with pretreatment cholesterol levels higher than 7.5 mmol/L and at least three coronary risk factors.[17] The cost-effectiveness of niacin in male patients aged 40 years with total cholesterol levels exceeding 6.9 mmol/L and one coronary risk factor has been estimated to be $14 900 dollars per life-year saved.[18] In the case of statin medications, the Scandinavian Simvastatin Survival Study (4S) demonstrated the ability of simvastatin, 20–40 mg daily, to reduce mortality by 30% in patients with a history of angina pectoris or acute myocardial infarction over a 5.4-year follow-up period.[19] Similarly, treatment with pravastatin, 40 mg per day, in patients with a history of unstable angina pectoris or myocardial infarction reduced mortality by 22%.[20] Economic analysis of the 4S study demonstrated that simvastatin therapy for male and female patients aged 59 years with serum cholesterol levels of 6.8 mmol/L resulted in a cost per life-year gained of $1600 and $4900, respectively, when considering direct and indirect costs.[21] Such figures would be considered highly cost-effective. For patients aged 35 years with established coronary heart disease and total cholesterol levels in the range 5.5–8.0 mmol/L, simvastatin therapy resulted in net savings.[21] Therefore statin therapy is considered to be highly cost-effective for many patients with angina pectoris. The benefit of statin therapy in patients with hyperlipidaemia but without angina pectoris has also been demonstrated.[22]

Conventional anti-anginal therapy

Current evidence supports the benefit of beta-blockade for patients with acute myocardial infarction. The evidence supporting the use of these drugs in unstable angina pectoris is based on limited data from randomized trials. A meta-analysis of studies involving 4700 patients with unstable angina demonstrated a 13% reduction in the risk of myocardial infarction among patients treated with beta-blockers. In view of the strong pathogenic link between unstable angina and acute myocardial infarction, current recommendations indicate that beta-blockers should be used as first-line agents in all acute coronary syndromes. Although the cost-effectiveness ratio of beta-blockade post myocardial infarction has been estimated to be approximately $5000 and $40 000 per life-year saved for high-risk and low-risk patients, respectively, data on the cost-effectiveness of beta-blockade in the treatment of stable angina pectoris are scarce.[23]

Like beta-blockers, nitrates are widely used in the management of angina pectoris, despite the lack of convincing data demonstrating that nitrates reduce either mortality or the rate of new myocardial infarction. Similarly, there are few data to demonstrate the cost-effectiveness of nitrate therapy in angina pectoris.

Coronary revascularization

Prior to the availability of coronary artery stenting, coronary artery bypass grafting was indicated for patients with unstable angina with a high-risk coronary artery anatomy (i.e. luminal obstruction of 50% or more of the left main coronary artery, or three-vessel disease with an associated reduction in the ejection fraction (less than 50%), or diabetes mellitus).[24] Meta-analysis of the randomized trials in which conventional angioplasty (PTCA) was compared with CABG in moderate-risk patients found no difference in terms of prognosis between these two strategies. However, patients undergoing PTCA had 10 times the risk of requiring repeated revascularization procedures and 1.6 times the risk of recurrent angina at 1 year.[25] In view of this, Hlatky et al.[26] investigated the quality of life, employment and medical care costs for 934 of the 1829 patients who were enrolled in the Bypass Angioplasty Revascularization Investigation (BARI) study over a 5-year follow-up period. Approximately two-thirds of the patients in the BARI study had unstable angina pectoris, and over half of them had previous myocardial infarction. The patients in the angioplasty group returned to work 5 weeks sooner, and the initial cost of angioplasty was 65% of the cost of surgery (i.e. $21 113 vs. $32 347). After 5 years, the total medical cost of angioplasty was 95% of the cost of surgery (i.e. $56 225 vs. $58 889). The higher cost of subsequent hospitalizations and cardiac medications accounted for the majority of costs in subsequent years in the angioplasty group.

The number of diseased vessels was the only baseline clinical factor with a significant influence on 4-year cumulative costs. The lowest cost was among patients with two-vessel disease in the angioplasty group ($52 930). The 5-year cost of angioplasty was significantly lower than that of surgery among patients with two-vessel disease ($52 930 vs. $58 498), but not among patients with three-vessel disease ($60 918 vs. $59 430). After a 5-year follow-up, the estimated cost-effectiveness ratio for surgery was $26 177 per year of life gained. Surgery appeared to be particularly cost-effective in treating patients with diabetes mellitus, because of their improved survival.[26]

Compared with PTCA alone, coronary artery stenting is associated with a higher rate of initial procedural success, a lower rate of restenosis at 6 months and a higher rate of event-free survival at 6 months. Abizaid et al. investigated the cost-effectiveness of coronary artery bypass grafting vs. PTCA plus stenting in diabetic patients with multi-vessel disease.[27] The authors estimated the incremental cost-effectiveness of coronary artery bypass grafting compared with stenting to be $20 947 in non-diabetic patients and $15 467 in diabetic patients. Disco *et al.* investigated the cost-effectiveness of CABG vs. per-cutaneous intervention in patients with multi-vessel disease.[28] These authors indicated that the effectiveness of CABG appeared to decrease with age, and this was not apparent for angioplasty with stenting. The incremental cost-effectiveness of CABG was $7750 for patients under 54 years of age, increasing to $48 117 for patients over 68 years of age. The authors concluded that coronary artery bypass grafting may remain the preferred treatment option for younger patients, whilst stenting becomes the more favourable option for older patients.

Summary

Management of angina pectoris may be expected to consume approximately 3% of the health-care budget. Identified variables with the greatest impact on expenditure include cardiovascular surgery, treatment in the general practice or hospital setting, number of years since the first diagnosis of angina, and whether the patient has stable or unstable angina pectoris. Treatment and prophylaxis with aspirin have been demonstrated to be cost-effective, as has the use of low-molecular-weight heparin (enoxaparin) in patients with unstable angina and non-Q-wave myocardial infarction. Appropriate selection of patients for therapy with glycoprotein IIb–IIIa receptor antagonists may prove cost-effective. Statin therapy reduces the requirement for revascularization procedures, and for some patients it leads to cost savings. Compared with PTCA, coronary artery bypass grafting appears to be cost-effective, particularly in patients with diabetes mellitus. The economic data indicate that CABG may remain the preferred treatment option for younger patients, whereas PTCA plus stenting is the more favourable option for older patients, in terms of medium-term cost analysis.

The costs associated with angina pectoris vary considerably from one country to another, and are in part related to differences in medical practice, percentage of gross national product spent on health, and the method of remuneration of practitioners. In general, costings are better described in communities where health care is paid for by way of patient insurance rather than in a state (especially monopolistic) system.

References

1. Wittels EH, Hay JW, Gotto AM. Medical costs of coronary artery disease. *Am J Cardiol* 1990; **65**: 432–40.

2. Andersson F, Kartman B. The cost of angina pectoris in Sweden. *Pharmacoeconomics* 1995; **8**: 233–44.

3. Russell MW, Huse DM, Drowns S *et al.* Direct medical costs of coronary artery disease in the United States. *Am J Cardiol* 1998; **81**: 110–15.

4. Kuntz KM, Fleischmann KE, Hunink M, Douglas PS. Cost-effectiveness of diagnostic strategies for patients with chest pain. *Ann Intern Med* 1999; **130**: 709–18.

5. Shaw LJ, Heller GV, Travin MI *et al.* Cost analysis of diagnostic testing for coronary artery disease in women with stable chest pain. Economics of Non-invasive Diagnosis (END) Study Group. *J Nucl Cardiol* 1999; **6**: 559–69.

6. Rask KJ, Deaton C, Culler SD *et al.* The effect of primary care gatekeepers on the management of patients with chest pain. *Am J Manag Care* 1999; **5**: 1274–82.

7. RISC Group. Risk of myocardial infarction and death during treatment with low-dose aspirin and intravenous heparin in men with unstable coronary artery disease (RISC). *Lancet* 1992; **336**: 827–30.

8. Juul-Moller S, Edvardsson N, John Matz B *et al.* Double-blind trial of aspirin in primary prevention of MI in patients with stable chronic angina pectoris. *Lancet* 1992; **340**: 1421–5.

9. Marissal J-P, Selke B, Lebrun T. Economic assessment of the secondary prevention of ischaemic events with lysine acetylsalicylate. *Pharmacoeconomics* 2000; **18**: 185–200.

10. Madar M, Berkowitz SD, Tcheng JE. Glycoprotein IIb/IIIa integrin blockade. *Circulation* 1998; **98**: 2629–35.

11. Heeschen C, Hamm CW, Heidenreich P. Costs and effectivity of treatment with tirofiban in patients with acute coronary syndromes: results from the PRISM trial. *Eur Heart J* 2000; **21 (Abstract Supplement)**: 478.

12. Houghton AR, Patel M, Hudson I. Cost implications of introducing the glycoprotein IIb/IIIa inhibitor tirofiban for the treatment of acute coronary syndromes on the coronary care unit. *Eur Heart J* 2000; **21 (Abstract Supplement)**: 219.

13. Detournay B, Huet X, Fagnani F, Montalescot G. Economic evaluation of enoxaparin sodium versus heparin in unstable angina. *Pharmacoeconomics* 2000; **18**: 83–9.

14. Mark DB, Cowper PA, Beckowitz S *et al.* Economic assessment of low-molecular-weight heparin (enoxaparin) versus unfractionated heparin in acute coronary syndrome patients: results from the ESSENCE randomised trial. *Circulation* 1998; **97**: 1702–7.

15. Fox KAA, Bosanquet N. Assessing the UK cost implications of the use of low-molecular-weight heparin in unstable coronary artery disease. *Br J Cardiol* 1998; **5**: 92–105.

16. Hay JW, Yu WM, Ashraf T. Pharmacoeconomics of lipid-lowering agents for primary and secondary prevention of coronary artery disease. *Pharmacoeconomics* 1999; **15**: 47–74.

17. Oster G, Epstein AM. Cost-effectiveness of antihyperlipidemic therapy in the prevention of coronary heart disease: the case of cholestyramine. *J Am Med Assoc* 1987; **258**: 2381–7.

18. Killey J. Hypercholesterolaemia: the cost of treatment in perspective. *South Med J* 1990; **83**: 1421–5.

19. Scandinavian Simvastatin Survival Study Group. Randomised trial of cholesterol lowering in 4444 patients with coronary heart disease: the Scandinavian Simvastatin Survival Study (4S). *Lancet* 1994; **344**: 1383–9.

20. LIPID Study Group. Prevention of cardiovascular events and death with pravastatin in patients with coronary heart disease and a broad range of initial cholesterol levels. *N Engl J Med* 1998; **339**: 1349–57.

21. Johannesson M, Jonsson B, Kjekshus J *et al.* Cost-effectiveness of simvastatin treatment to lower cholesterol levels in patients with coronary heart disease. *N Engl J Med* 1997; **336**: 332–6.

22. Shepherd J, Cobbe SM, Ford I *et al.* Prevention of coronary heart disease with pravastatin in men with hypercholesterolemia. *N Engl J Med* 1995; **333**: 1301–7.

23. Goldman L, Sia SB, Cook EF *et al.* Costs and effectiveness of routine therapy with long-term beta-adrenergic antagonists after myocardial infarction. *N Engl J Med* 1988; **319**: 152–7.

24. Bypass Angioplasty Revascularization Investigation (BARI) Investigators. Comparison of coronary bypass surgery with angioplasty in patients with multi-vessel disease. *N Engl J* Med 1996; **335**: 217–25.

25. Pocock SJ, Henderson RA, Richards AF *et al.* Meta-analysis of randomised trials comparing coronary angioplasty with bypass surgery. *Lancet* 1995; **346**: 1184–9.

26. Hlatky MA, Rogers WJ, Johnstone I *et al.* Medical care costs and quality of life after randomization to coronary angioplasty or coronary bypass surgery. *N Engl J Med* 1997; **336**: 92–9.

27. Abizaid A, Costa MA, Centemero M *et al.* Clinical and economic impact of diabetes mellitus on percutaneous and surgical treatment of multi-vessel coronary disease patients: insights from the Arterial Revascularization Therapy Study (ARTS) trial. *Circulation* 2001; **104**: 533–8.

28. Disco CMC, Lindeboom WK, Serruys PW *et al.* Comparison of effectiveness and cost effectiveness of CABG versus percutaneous intervention in patients with multi-vessel disease assessed by age. *Eur Heart J* 2000; **21 (Abstract 2567)**: 572.

Index